A Couple's Guide to Fertility

The Complete Sympto-Thermal Method

by

R. J. Huneger and Rose Fuller

Table of Contents

Abbreviation Glossary	v
Recommendation for Rules to Follow	vii
Introduction	1

CHAPTER ONE: THE SCIENCE BEHIND NFP

Male Fertility	5
Female Fertility	6
Menstrual Cycle	10
Reproductive Life and Categories	11

CHAPTER TWO: CHARTING THE SYMPTOMS

Waking Temperature	15
Tissue-Paper Examination	19
Vaginal Sensations	24
Peak Day	25
Cervical Sign	28
Secondary Signs	31

CHAPTER THREE: NFP GUIDELINES FOR AVOIDING

Basic Sympto-Thermal Rule	35
Relatively Infertile Time	
- 6-5-0 Day Rule	42
- Early Dry Days Rule	45
- Distinguishing Post-Intercourse Discharge	47
- Menses Fertile, Dry Days Infertile	48
- Earliest 6th Last Low Rule	49
- Short cut Approach	52
- Basic Mucus Rule	53
Temperature Only Rules	
- Mean Temperature Rule	56
- BBT Rule	58
Stress	59

CHAPTER FOUR: ACHIEVING PREGNANCY

Achieving and Identifying Pregnancy	61
Male Fertility Issues	65
Assisting Pregnancy	65
Emotional Issues	66

CHAPTER FIVE: SPECIAL CIRCUMSTANCES

Discontinuing Hormonal Contraceptives
- The Birth Control Pill and Patches   69
- Injectables ("The Shot")   71
- Implants   72
- Intrauterine Device   73

After Childbirth
- Miscarriage   75
- Not Breastfeeding   76
- Breastfeeding   76

Premenopause   82

CHAPTER SIX: COMMON QUESTIONS   85

CHAPTER SEVEN: BACKGROUND INFORMATION

Hormones   93
Menstrual Cycle Myths   94
Breast Self-Exam   95
Effectiveness   96
The Historical Foundations for NFP   98
High Tech NFP   99
Test Your Knowledge   100

CHAPTER EIGHT: LIVING WITH NATURAL FAMILY PLANNING

Natural Family Planning — "Natural"?   103
But Isn't This Just "Birth Control"?   106
What Does the Catholic Church Teach...?   108
Passing It On   115

ACKNOWLEDGMENTS

The diagrams of male and female anatomy on pages 4 and 6 and the menstrual cycle diagram on page 90 are reprinted with permission of the Human Life and Natural Family Planning Foundation. The cycle of seasons in nature and in the woman's cycle on pages 8 and 118 came from Gallagher, Heinzen, Hogan, Taylor, *Teaching Catholic Family Values: A Parent Handbook*, Leaflet Missal Company, 1996. The cover was designed by Sean Fuller.

Thanks to Dr. Josef Roetzer, Elisabeth Roetzer, and Karen Tuerck of INER and Holly Denman for assistance with the 1991 edition. Gail Hitchcock assisted with proofreading the 1997 edition. Dr. Bernharda Meyer and Janet McLaughlin helped with excellent comments in the 1991 and 1997 edition. Janet McLaughlin provided detailed assistance in the development of the 2004 edition. Lauren Fuller provided excellent comments in the 2009 edition.

All rights reserved. This book, or parts thereof, may not be reproduced in any form without prior written permission from the publisher, Northwest Family Services.
Revised edition, March 2004.

© 1978, 1979, 1980, 1981, 1983, 1985, 1986, 1991, 1997, 1999, 2002, 2004, 2006, 2009 Northwest Family Services, R. J. Huneger

ISBN #1-880220-00-8

All rights reserved. No part of this publication may be reproduced or transmitted in any form or by any means electronic or mechanical, including photography, recording, or any information storage and retrieval system now known or to be invented, without written permission from the publisher.

Printed in the U.S.A.
Northwest Family Services
6200 SE King Road, Portland, Oregon 97222
Telephone: (503) 546-6377, FAX (503) 546-9397
website: www.nwfs.org
email: service@nwfs.org
Online NFP instruction is available at www.nwfs.org

FOREWORD

Currently there is an increasing interest in Natural Family Planning around the world. And a large number of programs and published materials promoting Natural Family Planning are now within reach of the general public. Not all of the available materials, however, make it clear that there are a variety of methodologies that can be used singly or in combination to meet the needs and preferences of couples in various circumstances and with diverse backgrounds. It is a special feature of this manual with accompanying instruction program that it provides the most comprehensive information possible on different approaches to natural family planning.

With continuing interest I have observed how this manual and the related materials have been compiled during the last few years, during which information from all the available literature, as well as the practical experience of the teaching and learning couples who helped to develop this material, were incorporated into the present work.

It is a pleasure for me to recommend this new edition of the entire set of client and teaching materials to all those who wish to obtain comprehensive information regarding Natural Family Planning, in particular because the material itself is continuously revised and kept up to date.

Josef Roetzer, M.D., November 1, 1981

It is a joy to commend the 1991 edition of this manual to the reader, who may be unaware of how this book has over and over again proven its value to so many couples, and been adopted in many places in the United States as the basis for local Natural Family Planning program services. The most recent developments in the field have once again been incorporated into this handbook and the program of instruction associated with it.

Josef Roetzer, M.D., June 10, 1991

Abbreviation Glossary

BBT Basal Body Temperature.

BMR Basic Mucus Rule.

BT Breast Tenderness.

CIT Completely Infertile Time. The post-ovulatory phase of the cycle which begins when the Sympto-Thermal Rule is fulfilled. The CIT lasts through the end of the cycle, ending when menstruation begins.

EDDR Early Dry Days Rule. Infertility may be assumed at the end of the day once you are sure you were dry all day first, by all the signs you checked, and you have a history of consistently observing a change in your signs on or before the 6th last low temperature.

FTSL Full Thermal Shift Level.

IP Intermenstrual Pain. A sharp pain or crampiness, usually noticed only for a few hours. May be associated with ovulation.

LAM Lactational Amenorrhea Method.

NFP Natural Family Planning.

PFT Possibly Fertile Time. The phase of the cycle assumed to be fertile. Ovulation occurs during this phase of the cycle.

PK Peak Day. The last day of the most fertile sign (usually EW-M or L).

PRB Pre-Rise Baseline.

RIT Relatively Infertile Time. Day 1 of the cycle begins with bright red bleeding and is the first day of the pre-ovulatory time of the cycle, which continues until the first day of possible fertility according to the rule a couple is applying.

STR Sympto-Thermal Rule. Identifies the onset of the CIT.

NATURAL FAMILY PLANNING:
Learner Assignments

A Note to the Reader:
This manual provides essential background in the basics needed to observe and chart naturally occurring signs of fertility. It is recommended that before applying the information to your own situation you work in conjunction with a certified NFP Provider competent in the Sympto-Thermal Method of NFP.

1. Participate in all classes, on time, as a couple (if possible), and check your understanding by successfully doing the learning activities.

2. Turn in copies of your charts to your NFP Provider for the first six cycles and show you know how to apply the guidelines to them. Start charting right away.

After Session One:
Read Chapter One: introduction, anatomy and physiology (pages 5-13). Chapter Three: establishing the Pre-Rise Baseline (pages 36-37). Chapter Two: waking temperature, tissue paper exam, vaginal sensations, and Peak Day (pages 15-27). Use the Beginner Chart (with instructions) to chart temperature and tissue.

After Session Two:
Read about cervical and secondary signs (pages 28-32) and Chapter Seven: effectiveness (pages 96-97). Achieving pregnancy is covered in Chapter Three. Chapter Four: Basic Sympto-Thermal Rule and 6-5-0 Day Rule (pages 35-44) and Chapter Eight: Living With NFP (pages 103-115). Think about it. Talk about it. Read the handouts provided in class.

After Session Three:
Read all of Chapter Three, especially about assuming infertility beyond Day 6 (pages 45-52), and the Basic Mucus Rule (pages 53-55), along with Chapter Six: Common Questions (pages 85-91). For the next six months send in your chart at the end of each cycle.

Note: All Charts found in this text are identified by a number in the upper left hand corner.

Recommendations for Rules to Follow:

Your NFP Provider will make recommendations after you have started charting. Circle the rules recommended by your Provider and then review the guideline as needed.

1. Abstain and chart

Completely Infertile Time
2. Sympto-Thermal Rule (p. 35)
3. Mean Temperature Rule (p. 56)
4. BBT Rule (p. 58)
5. Other:_____

Relatively Infertile Time
6. Abstain
7. Menses fertile, dry days afterward infertile (p. 48)
8. 6-5-0 Day Rule (p. 42)
9. Earliest 6th Last Low Temperature Rule (p. 49)
10. Early Dry Days Rule (p. 45):
    a) Tissue
    b) Sensation
    c) Cervix: F.L.C.Ø.
11. Discharge after Intercourse (p. 47)
    a) Non-consecutive dry evenings.
    b) F.L.C.Ø. cervix before intercourse.
12. Basic Mucus Rule/Activity 10 (p. 53)
13. Basic Mucus Rule/Patch Rule/Activity 11 (p. 79)
14. Basic Infertile Pattern/Cycling, Activity 12
    a) First change
    b) Borderline = day_____
    c) Peak + 4
15. Basic Infertile Pattern/Not Cycling, Activity 13
16. When in doubt during the Relatively Infertile Time, assume as if EW-M and count Pk+4.
17. All bleeding other than true menses is considered fertile, as if EW-M; apply a Pk+4 count.
18. Special cases:
    a) Intensive Breastfeeding, weeks 1 to 12 postpartum (p. 76)
    b) Post-Peak stretch as if "M," (p. 40)
19. Achieving (p. 61)
    a) Use days of the best quality/quantity EW-M until the first high temperature.
    b) After 6-12 cycles, seek medical evaluation.

INTRODUCTION

Did you ever have the notion that fertility is so unpredictable and confusing that it is impossible to understand or manage? Can you imagine being able to avoid or achieve a pregnancy — naturally? Wouldn't it be nice to know enough about your fertility to know when something wasn't quite right and to ask intelligent questions about it? This is all possible by learning Natural Family Planning (NFP). Couples learning NFP liken it to taking a course in themselves. NFP is using the knowledge of the man's and woman's fertility to avoid or achieve a pregnancy based on the couple's family planning intention. They begin by understanding basic observation and charting skills. The next step is learning how to interpret the observations. As a result, they know where they are in the cycle regardless of the woman's cycle length.

The NFP method discussed in this book is known as the Sympto-Thermal Method (STM). It recognizes that each woman has several observable body signs which relate to her fertile and infertile times. These signs reflect hormonal changes in the menstrual cycle. The cervical mucus flow, and vaginal sensations, and changes at the cervix tell when fertility is beginning, and when it is greatest; the temperature rise afterward confirms that the fertile time has ended.

> "Chastity is one of the greatest disciplines without which the mind cannot attain requisite firmness." Ghandi

Learning about couple fertility makes it easier to appreciate periodic abstinence as a way of avoiding pregnancy. Fertility is "periodic" — there is a definite fertile time each cycle which can be identified — but most of the cycle is infertile. Couples can know when a particular act of intercourse is likely to lead to pregnancy, and it can be identified early on.

One basic aspect of NFP is that it is based on fertility acceptance instead of fertility suppression. It starts from the idea that the power to transmit life is not a disease, but a wonderful gift, to be respected in its integrity. Mother Teresa of Calcutta called periodic abstinence "self-control out of love." The decision neither to harm nor to suppress fertility calls forth a decision to love your spouse wholeheartedly. Where this love is strong, the sacrifice of periodic abstinence is a welcome (though sometimes difficult) challenge to keep true love alive in many ways in marriage.

There can be some unexpected side effects found with the use of NFP. Some couples say that the greatest benefit of NFP is not that it is effective for avoiding or achieving pregnancy but that it is a touchstone, calling for the same traits in the area of family planning that are fundamental for marriage as a whole. It becomes a barometer of love.

Some say NFP is the best kept secret around. Others wonder why more people don't select NFP; after all, it has no negative side effects. Why do couples choose NFP?

Many people are concerned about the types of foods they eat, the need for exercise, and the environment which surrounds them. For example, one woman, while tending her organic garden, suddenly wonders why she is putting chemicals (the Pill) into her body daily which she would never add to her compost pile. A husband, after reading the Pill insert and learning about all the possible complications, tells his wife there has to be something better. He wants her off the Pill because he is justifiably concerned about the side effects. Another woman, attentive to her physical appearance, doesn't shed those last ten pounds until she is free of artificial hormones. These people recognize that such factors impact the quality of their lives and their relationships.

Some couples are looking for an effective alternative to artificial birth control — they may be tired of "suiting up for intercourse" by using condoms, diaphragms, or spermicides. The notion of "protecting" oneself from a spouse may seem contrary to the notion of marital fidelity. Other couples are coming to know about the abortifacient potential of hormonal contraceptives such as the Pill, injectables, and implants and devices like the IUD, and may turn to NFP out of reverence for life itself.

All of these people, in varying degrees, begin to appreciate how NFP is consistent in all areas of life. A holistic perspective of the human person is revealed in the sensitive subject of sexuality and fertility. Respecting the normal fertility processes with the practice of NFP conveys a consistent message about the whole array of sexual issues and personal responsibility.

It is no longer uncommon to hear couples say that they have heard about and want to share in the marriage-building elements in NFP: mutual responsibility and increased communication in the area of sexuality and marriage as a whole. Over seventy percent of couples responding to the Northwest Family Services 12-month follow-up questionnaire indicate that using NFP has increased their communication level. Other studies have shown that couples who use NFP have a greater spiritual intimacy than their contracepting peers.

Some people wonder if periodic abstinence will result in disharmony in their relationship. A five-country study conducted by the World Health Organization asked couples who used NFP if marital friction resulted, and 80 to 99 percent indicated it was uncommon. It is true that the sacrifice associated with periodic abstinence is counter-cultural; the inherent sexual tension reportedly helps keep intimacy alive in a marriage.

When people learn about the advantages, many of them are interested. For example, about 750 women were randomly selected as part of a phone survey. The women were given a brief description of NFP including the ability to use the information to either achieve or avoid a pregnancy. While only 2.8% were current users of NFP and about the only knowledge the other women had was a notion of Calendar Rhythm, 22.5% of the women said they were likely to use NFP in the future to avoid a pregnancy and 37.4% said they would use it to achieve a pregnancy.[1] On another note, a cohort of physicians were asked about their knowledge of NFP. The majority of physicians underestimated the effectiveness of NFP equating it with Calendar Rhythm.[2]

---

1. Stanford, J., et al, "Women's Interest in Natural Family Planning," *The Journal of Family Practice*, Vol. 46, No. 1 (Jan) 1998.
2. Stanford, J., et al, "Physicians' Knowledge and Practices Regarding Natural Family Planning," *Obstetrics & Gynecology*, Vol. 94, No. 5, November 1999.

NFP can significantly impact the couple's relationship on all levels. For example, one couple said, "We've been put in a position where our intimacy level in all parts of our relationship (spiritual, emotional, marital) are put in front of us. It has caused us to grow and learn more about each other's self-esteem and security specifically in the area of sexuality, but it has carried over into all areas of our life." Even though self-control can be a challenge, men and women alike speak about the increased self-respect they experience in being able to manage their sexual feelings.

NFP is also sought by couples seeking to live in accord with their Church's teaching against artificial birth control, or because of an informed commitment to follow the principles which are the basis for their Church's teachings.

Most couples come not for just one, but for a combination of the above reasons. In time, it becomes for them a "way of life." All in all, NFP is a lesson in self-understanding — an opportunity to know more about yourself and your spouse.

Chastity within marriage refers to the ability or strength to integrate one's sexual feelings and actions according to what is truly best for oneself and one's spouse. With that understanding, these words of Indian author Rabindranath Tagore have a special application in NFP: "Chastity is a wealth that comes from an abundance of love."

> "The great danger for family life, in the midst of any society whose idols are pleasure, comfort and independence, lies in the fact that people close their hearts and become selfish."
> **Pope John Paul II**

CHAPTER ONE: THE SCIENCE BEHIND NFP

There is a sound scientific basis to modern Natural Family Planning. NFP requires no drugs, devices, or surgical procedures, yet is effective for achieving or avoiding a pregnancy. Understanding a few basics about anatomy and physiology will help you to understand the scientific foundations of NFP.

Male Fertility

It is often said that the brain is the primary sex organ. This statement is certainly true when thinking of the hormonal processes that direct fertility. The intricate process of male fertility is initiated from the pituitary gland, which is attached to the brain. Hormonal messengers are sent from the pituitary gland to the *testes* (testicles) inside the scrotum. The scrotum is a baggy pouch of skin resting beneath the penis. The

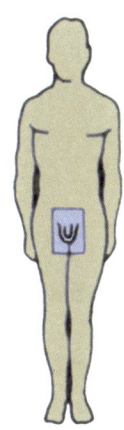
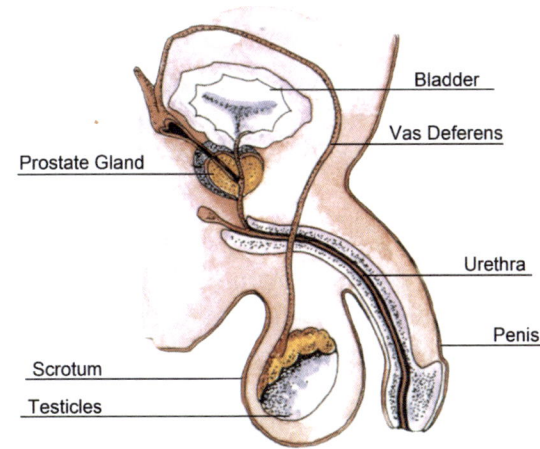

testes, the male sex glands, produce testosterone, the hormone responsible for male body characteristics, and sperm, the male sex cell.

Once puberty is reached, a man begins producing sperm constantly. Sperm cells need a temperature slightly lower than the normal body temperature to survive; thus, the need for the testicles to be outside of the main body area. The *scrotum* functions to maintain the proper temperature.

Semen, which is a thick, white substance observed in an ejaculation, is composed of sperm cells and seminal fluid. Most men produce millions of sperm a day with the average being between 100-200 million sperm daily. Sperm cells take about 10 weeks to fully mature. The developing sperm cells are transported from the testes to the epididymis where the cells become capable of moving. The sperm cells remain in the epididymis until the time of ejaculation. When the sperm cells leave the epididymis, they travel through a tube called the vas deferens, which joins with the urethra. In this tube, the sperm cells are mixed with fluids from the prostate gland, the seminal vesicles, and Cowper's gland. Again, the mixture of sperm cells and seminal fluid is called semen.

The *penis* is made of spongy tissue which becomes erect during sexual arousal. During ejaculation, the semen is released through the urethra, a tube in the center of the penis. Semen is mostly seminal fluid and contains millions of sperm (a cubic centimeter of it may contain 20- to 500-million sperm), with a high concentration of sperm being in the very first part of the ejaculate to leave the penis. The pre-ejaculatory secretions also contain sperm. These secretions may leave the penis without the man being conscious of it. Sperm also can be discharged from the penis in urine or be flushed from the reproductive system during nocturnal emission (wet dream). Both urine and semen pass through the urethra in the penis, but a valve between the prostate gland and the bladder closes to prevent urine from being released when semen is ejaculated.

A mature, healthy man develops hundreds of thousands of sperm cells every day. Sperm cells are extremely small. It has been said that all the sperm needed to produce the next generation of Americans could be placed on the head of a pin. Even a minute quantity of semen can cause pregnancy.

Key Points:
· A healthy man produces sperm continuously and is always fertile.
· Genital contact when the woman is fertile may result in pregnancy.

Female Fertility

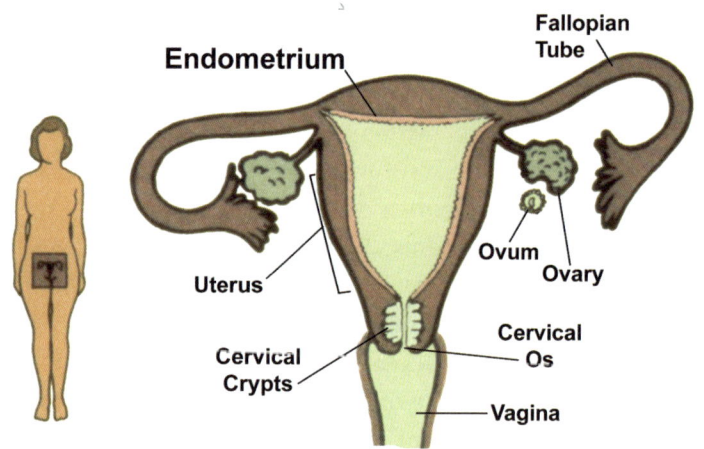

In contrast to the man, the woman's reproductive organs lie inside her body. This is a protective mechanism to ensure the safety of the unborn child as he or she develops within the mother. A woman's fertility (her ability to become pregnant) is also different in that it is not continuous. The couple is potentially fertile for about 7 to 10 days of the cycle.

The woman's fertility is orchestrated from the pituitary gland. It releases hormones on a cyclic basis which stimulate the ovaries to release an egg cell. The delicate interplay results in what is known as the menstrual cycle. The menstrual cycle begins with the first day of bright red blood flow which is called the menstrual *period* or menses. The menstrual period normally lasts 4 to 7 days. The typical menstrual *cycle* is between 23 and 40 days long. The cycle length counted from the first day of the menstrual period until the day before the next period begins. The entire menstrual cycle is focused around the event of ovulation; that is, the day the woman releases a mature ovum or egg cell. The woman is fertile for a short time during her menstrual cycle, and this fertile time is observable through a variety of signs.

Whereas the man begins producing sperm at puberty, the woman's ovaries already contained at birth all the *ova* (eggs) she will ever have — up to 200,000 ova. At puberty, these ova begin to mature. In response to hormone signals, an *ovum* (egg) is released from the ovary during ovulation. The *fallopian tubes* are the passageways from the ovaries to the uterus. At the ends of the fallopian tubes are fimbria, fingerlike projections, which catch and transport the egg toward the uterus (womb). The *uterus* is about the size of a small pear, but is very elastic and expands greatly during pregnancy to accommodate the baby. The *endometrium* (the inner lining of the uterus) is renewed each cycle to prepare for pregnancy. The bottom part of the uterus is the *cervix*. Pockets of cells called *cervical crypt*s line the cervix. These cells produce a special fluid called cervical mucus which occurs around the time of ovulation. The *cervical os* is the "mouth" or opening of the cervix. The vagina is a muscular tube that receives the penis during intercourse, serves as a birth canal, and allows menstrual fluid and cervical mucus to pass to the outside of the body.

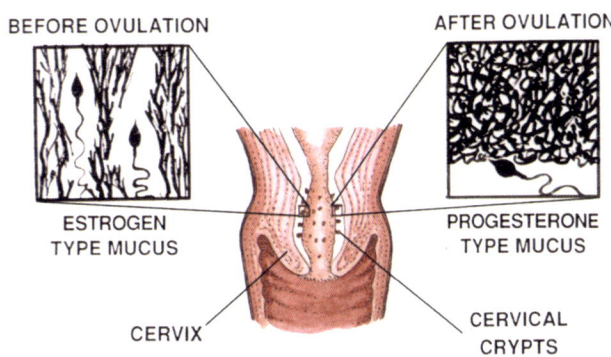

On one day each cycle, about two weeks before menstruation, ovulation occurs. Usually only one egg cell is released. If more than one is released, such as is the case with fraternal twins, the second ovulation will occur within the same 24-hour time span. The egg dies within 24 hours or less if not fertilized by a sperm. The woman is fertile for several more days because of the cervical mucus.

Several days *before* ovulation the cervical crypts produce a special fertility mucus. The woman may both *see* and *feel* the cervical mucus. During the course of her menstrual cycle, a woman usually experiences a transition from dry days to mucus days back to dry days again. To understand the observable changes the woman notices, it sometimes helps to review the microscopic changes. The diagram shown above displays the microscopic structure of the cervical mucus at its two extremes: Type E (estrogen type) and Type G (progesterone type). Type G cervical mucus is dense and thicket-like, resulting in a biological barrier at the cervix. Usually, women observe dryness when Type G cervical mucus is present.

Type E cervical mucus has a ladder-like structure resulting in a stretchability property called "Spinnbarkeit," and it forms a "ferning" pattern if dried and viewed with a microscope.[3] Type E cervical mucus also filters out abnormal sperm cells, allowing the healthiest sperm into the reproductive tract. This fertility mucus forms channels that direct sperm cells upwards to the uterus. This type of cervical mucus creates a friendly environment for sperm.

		Couple Fertility	
Man	Sperm	Sperm +	Sperm
Woman's Cycle		Egg + Cervical Mucus	

---

3. For a detailed analysis of Type G and Type E (with its several subtypes – mainly L and S) read "The Discovery of Different Types of Cervical Mucus and the Billings Ovulation Method," by Professor Erik Odeblad, http://www.woomb.org/omrrca/bulletin/vol21/no3/discovery.shtml.

Type E cervical mucus is a signal of impending ovulation. As the follicle (early egg cell) develops before ovulation, it releases estrogen which causes the cervical os to open and the cervical mucus to change in quality, quantity, and consistency, becoming more alkaline, clearer, and stretchy with a distinct slippery and lubricative quality. The cervical mucus is the reason that the fertile time of the cycle starts several days before ovulation. Sperm survival is assisted with the quality of the mucus. Sperm usually die within hours in the acidic environment of the vagina. With the presence of good cervical mucus the sperm can live 3 to 5 days.

Natural Family Planning is based on the often overlooked fact that fertility is always "couple fertility": it takes both a man and a woman to conceive a child. Human behavior, as well as biology, is involved. Biologically, fertility requires sperm from the man and an egg and cervical mucus from the woman. The woman is the reason the couple is fertile only part of the cycle.

If intercourse occurs when the cervical mucus is clear, stretchy, or lubricative, sperm can live as long as 3 to 5 days. This means there can be a time lag of several days between intercourse and conception — for example, intercourse on Monday could, under certain conditions, result in conception on Friday. Conception, also called fertilization, almost always occurs in the fallopian tube when the sperm and egg unite; this is when the new human life begins.

Once ovulation has occurred, the housing that the egg was released from becomes a corpus luteum or "yellow body" in the ovary. The corpus luteum secretes the hormone progesterone. Progesterone has several important effects.

1. Ovulation is prevented.

Progesterone works immediately to prevent a further ovulation. When progesterone is present, the pituitary will no longer signal for the development of follicles or ovulation. If another egg is released, this must be within a 24-hour time span. Once ovulation occurs, the woman will soon be infertile.

2. Preparation for a possible pregnancy.

Progesterone enriches the lining of the uterus, to prepare it to receive new life, in case pregnancy should occur. ("Pro-gesterone" means pro-gestation or favoring pregnancy.)

3. Cervical mucus dries up.

Progesterone causes the cervical mucus to thicken and form an impenetrable biological plug preventing sperm, bacteria, and other organisms from entering into the uterine environment.

4. Temperature rises.

Progesterone causes the woman's waking temperature (also known as basal body temperature) to rise to a higher level and remain high.

The life span of the corpus luteum is about two weeks. When it stops functioning, the uterine lining collapses and menstruation occurs. When a woman becomes pregnant, human chorionic gonadotropin (HCG) is secreted from her baby's placenta to sustain the pregnancy. With pregnancy, the woman's temperature remains high and she doesn't experience a menstrual period.

Analogy to the Seasons

It is sometimes helpful to relate the woman's fertility cycle to the changing seasons of the year. Menstruation is likened to autumn with the falling leaves. The dry days relate to the barren winter. Spring time brings forth new life and reminds us that the days of cervical mucus are fertile days. Summer time is when the air is warmer and relates to the high temperature phase. This analogy is further developed in the following manner. If a seed is planted during the dry season, it will not geminate. But if planted during the wet season, there will be a harvest. And, in between the dry and wet seasons, sometimes there is enough moisture for a seed to germinate.

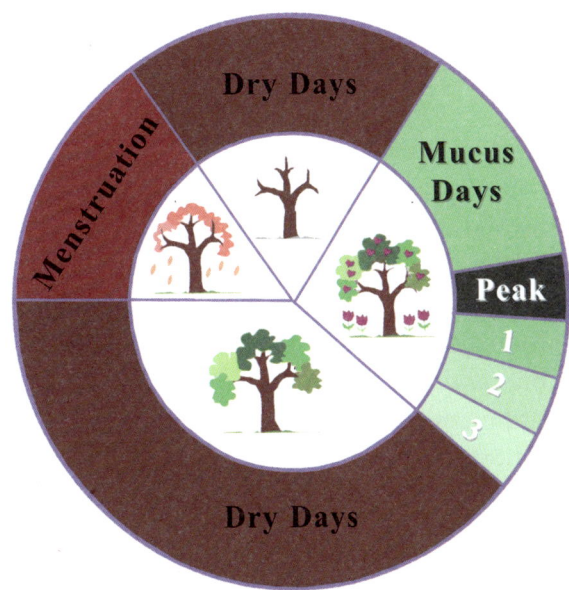

The Seasons of the Cycle

are like the Seasons of the Year

Key Points:

- Ovulation occurs on one day each cycle about two weeks before the next menstrual period.
- All eggs are released within a single 24-hour time period.
- The egg dies within 24 hours if not fertilized by sperm.
- If good cervical mucus is present, sperm can live 3 to 5 days.

The Menstrual Cycle

Many people believe the menstrual cycle is almost always 28 days in length and that ovulation always occurs on Day 14. The majority of women, however, do not consistently have 28-day cycles or ovulate on Day 14. For a given woman, the length of the menstrual cycle varies from one cycle to the next. It is not uncommon for a woman to have a cycle range difference of about a week or so between her shortest and longest cycles. In a given woman, for example, cycles ranging from 27-34 days may be noticed over a one-year time span.

Cycle Length

When speaking about the menstrual cycle, the time that varies is the time before ovulation. It can be affected by age, stress and the reproductive category. The time before ovulation is like an accordion and can be long one cycle and short the next. The time after ovulation is like a straightedge and is fairly constant from one cycle to the next in a given woman. This is the time of the cycle that is about two weeks long.

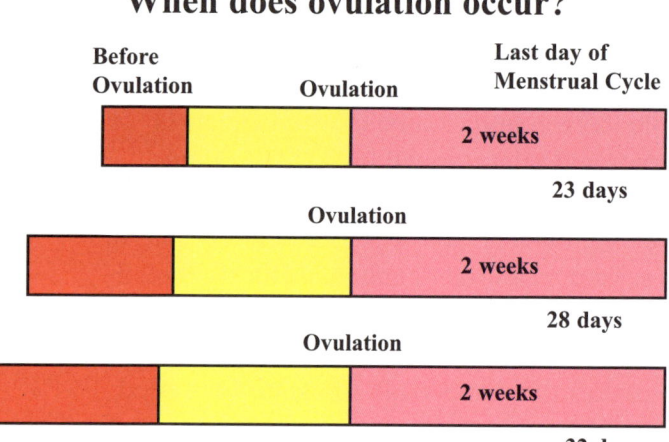

NFP Cycle Phases

For purposes of NFP, the cycle has three phases: the pre-ovulatory "*Relatively Infertile Time*," the ovulatory "*Possibly Fertile Time*," and the post-ovulatory "*Completely Infertile Time*." Pre-ovulatory infertility is called "Relative Infertility" because the body is again preparing for ovulation. The Relatively Infertile Time begins with the first day of bright red blood flow and extends until the start of fertility. This is the time of the cycle with the greatest variability in length.

The fertile time is called "Possibly Fertile" because even intercourse during the known fertile time does not always result in a pregnancy. Ovulation occurs somewhere during the Possibly Fertile Time, but we cannot pinpoint any day as the day of ovulation. The Possibly Fertile Time is identified by observing cervical mucus signs as well as the cervix. The end of this time is determined by the changing mucus pattern and a sustained temperature rise.

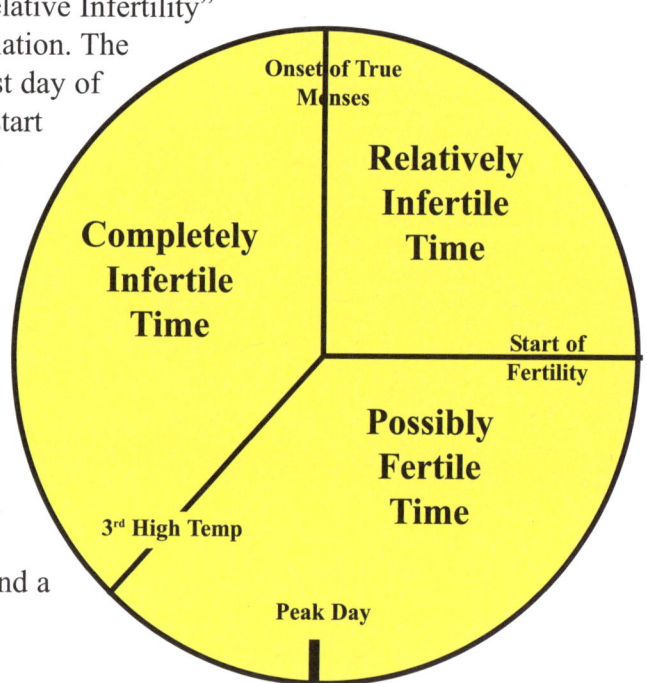

Finally, the time after ovulation is known as "Completely Infertile" because ovulation is no longer possible this cycle. This time of the cycle is determined with a sustained temperature pattern and a change away from the most fertile sign.

Periodic Abstinence

Natural Family Planning prevents pregnancy when the couple abstains during the fertile time. That is why NFP is sometimes called "periodic abstinence." "Abstinence" means complete abstinence: not only must full intercourse be avoided, but also all genital contact. When the woman is fertile, pregnancy can result from mere contact of the penis with the vaginal opening, even without penetration or ejaculation (and even if contraceptive measures are taken). This is referred to as "genital contact." Any means by which sperm can be conveyed to the vaginal opening, such as hand-to-genital contact or soaking through clothing touching the vagina, can possibly result in pregnancy, while the woman is fertile.

Also, the use of barrier contraceptives during the fertile time can confuse the use of NFP, one should expect to experience the typical pregnancy rates of the products used. For example, while perfect use of the condom is 98 percent, the typical pregnancy rate is 86 percent. That means that out of a 100 women using the condom as their means of birth control, 14 will experience an unintended pregnancy. In addition, some couples may be less vigilant in their use of NFP if they come to rely on contraceptives as well. This would, of course, reduce the overal effectiveness of the method.

Reproductive Life and Categories

There are two other factors which influence the cycle length: the woman's gynecological age (the number of years since her first menstrual period) and her reproductive category. The menstrual cycle more or less reflects everyday life, but it also reflects the stage of the reproductive lifetime a woman is in. All people have a chronological age (from birth). Women also have a gynecological age which is from menarche – that is, from the first menstrual period on.

During the woman's reproductive lifetime she will experience three phases:

The Woman's Reproductive Life: 3 Stages (Rudolf Vollman, *The Menstrual Cycle*, 1977.)		
Adolescence	*Maturity*	*Premenopause*
• First 5-8 years after menarche. • Cycles are generally longer, quite variable. • This is a time of growing toward prime fertility.	• About 20-30 years long. • Cycles are generally shorter, more regular. • Cycles are usually ovulatory, almost every cycle (almost all cycles show a sustained temperature rise during maturity).	• Last 5-8 years before menopause. • Cycles are generally longer, quite variable. • Fertility decreases as a woman ovulates fewer and fewer cycles, i.e., shows more and more flat patterns between bleedings.

Adolescence and premenopause are times of transition in a woman's life. During adolescence women move toward their greatest time of fertility, and from age 35 through menopause the woman's fertility decreases dramatically. Because cycle variation is "normal" during adolescence and premenopause, there is no need to "treat" it with hormones. In other words, women don't need to experience a bleeding every 28 days to be normal. Another transition time is post-childbirth. "Irregular" cycles may occur as the body is settling back into its previous cycling pattern.

Though there is a great deal of variation in cycle length among all women, a given woman can easily come to learn her own cycle pattern. During the mature years, the cycle length is consistent for most women. Reproductive categories are a useful way to understand different cycling situations women experience. For purposes of NFP, a given reproductive category relates to a specific set of guidelines. Let's review ten different reproductive categories.

Reproductive Category	Cycle Pattern	Additional Comments
Typical	Cycles are always 23 to 40 days long.	
Non-Typical: a) Short b) Long	a) Some cycles are 22 days or shorter. b) Some cycles are more than 40 days long.	This category does not include cycle variations caused by stress, discontinuation of hormones, or childbirth.
Premenopause	Cycles can be variable in length.	Women who are 45 years or older, or earlier if there is a family history of early menopause, or if she has symptoms of premenopause before age 45.
Achieving (difficulty conceiving)	Cycles can appear typical or be quite variable.	Couple has tried to achieve a pregnancy unsuccessfully for 6 or more cycles.
Pregnant	No menstrual periods.	
Post-Hormonal	Variable cycle pattern, in some cases a complete absence of menstruation.	
Post-Miscarriage	Cycles usually return quickly to the woman's typical pattern.	
Intensive Breastfeeding	No menstrual periods.	Specific definition, see page 76
Breastfeeding, not yet cycling	No menstrual periods.	
Not Breastfeeding, not yet cycling	No menstrual periods.	

Key Points:
- The menstrual cycle typically varies in length from cycle to cycle with about a week or so difference between the shortest and longest cycle.
- The high temperature phase (luteal phase) lasts about two weeks, and this length is constant from cycle to cycle.
- Women experience three reproductive phases: adolescence, maturity, and premenopause.
- Women can experience a variety of reproductive categories (e.g., childbirth) which will impact their cycles and the application of NFP.

CHAPTER TWO: CHARTING THE SYMPTOMS

The Waking Temperature

If you have ever thought that your body temperature is a constant 98.6°F, try taking your temperature at different times of the day, and you will notice fluctuations. The body's temperature changes throughout the day, with the lowest, more consistent temperature being earliest in the morning. These temperature fluctuations are due to circadian rhythms (an internal biological clock), not merely to increased activity. These variables are notable when people experience what is commonly called "jet lag." Women who use NFP can capture reliable information by observing their "basal body temperature." "Basal" means the body temperature at rest, unaffected by any activity. It will be referred to as the "waking temperature" because it is taken immediately upon waking from rest.

A fertile woman who takes her waking temperature daily under the same conditions will notice a biphasic pattern during her cycle. "Biphasic" means it has two levels. First, a *lower* level lasts from menstruation until about the time of ovulation. Then, there is a rise to a *higher* level where it remains high until the end of the cycle. Ovulation occurs within a few days before or after the rise to an overall higher level. We can't pinpoint any day on the temperature curve as being exactly when ovulation occurs. Some ask if the "dip" that sometimes occurs in the temperature pattern before the rise pinpoints "the day" of ovulation — no, the dip is not an accurate indicator of ovulation.

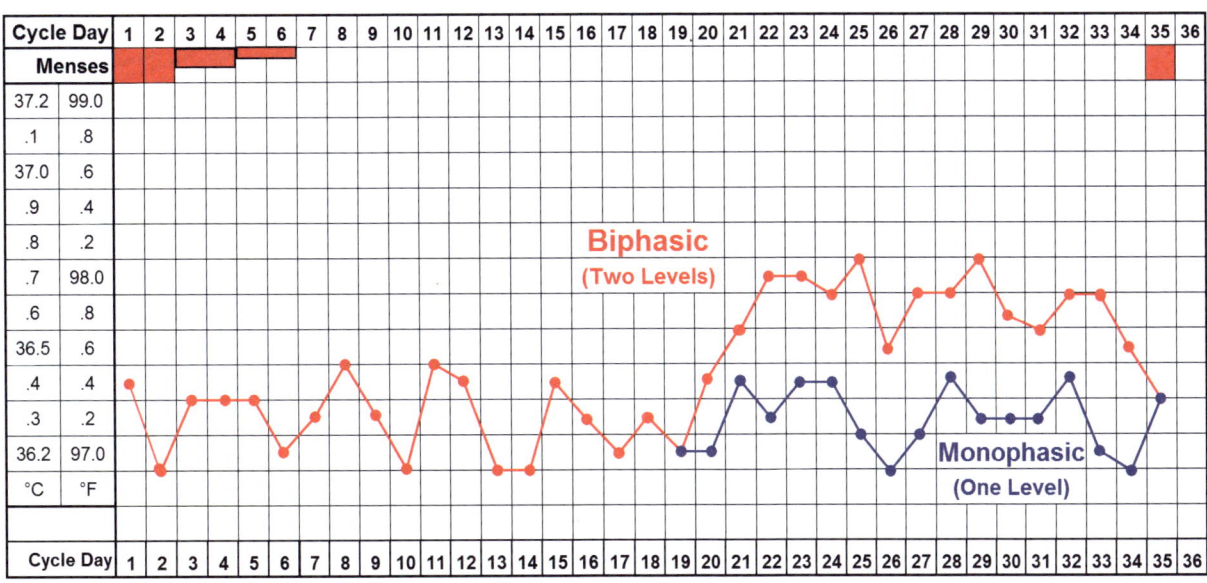

The significance of the temperature rise is that you know:
- When the post-ovulatory infertile time is beginning. The bleeding one to two weeks later is really menstruation.
- You are most likely pregnant once the temperature is high for 18-20 days.
- You are probably not ovulating if you have a "monophasic pattern"; that is, only one level, never showing a rise during intervals between bleeding.

Temperature-Taking Techniques

The difference between the low and the high temperature levels is only about one-half a degree Fahrenheit, so you must take your temperature properly. The best way to do so is by using a digital thermometer which registers in 0.1°F. Some people ask about the use of "ear thermometers" (tympanic thermometers) for NFP. These thermometers are not accurate enough for NFP purposes nor are glass fever thermometers.

Glass basal body thermometers have traditionally been used with NFP; however, we now use digital 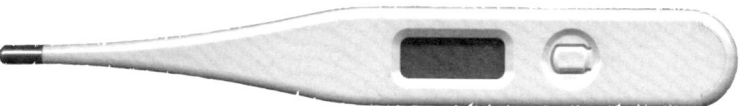 thermometers for environmental reasons. One can obtain an accurate temperature with a digital thermometer. Your digital thermometer should have a "recall" button to retrieve the reading later and read out temperatures to within 0.1°F from 96 –100°F [to within 0.05°C from 35.7–37.7°C]. It is recommended you continue taking your temperature for an additional minute beyond the "beep," as the temperature usually is not done registering until that point. If you compare one thermometer with another the overall pattern will be the same; however, the exact readings may not match.

Take good care of your thermometer

Clean your digital thermometer with warm, soapy water or ethyl alcohol, being careful not to immerse it in water or boil it. Make sure water does not get into the display panel or the power switch.

If you use a glass mercury-based thermometer, be sure to keep it away from excess heat. Don't leave it on or near a heater. If you are on a trip, don't put it in the car glove compartment or anywhere else in the car where heat can build up. Wash it with rubbing alcohol or cool water. It is necessary to shake the thermometer to move the mercury to a lower level. Be sure to shake it down over a soft surface, like your bed, in case it slips from your hand. If you suspect a fever, use an ordinary thermometer. If you break a mercury-based thermometer, please check with your local poison control for proper disposal procedures.

Methods for Temperature Taking

There are three good methods of taking your waking temperature: oral, vaginal, and rectal. Don't use readings taken from under the armpit or with the ear method; these methods are not accurate enough for NFP use.

Using a digital thermometer, take your temperature for about 2 minutes. This is about a minute beyond the "beep" indicating the initial reading has been reached. This extended time increases the accuracy of the reading. If you are using a glass thermometer, please take your temperature for 5-8 minutes.

- The *Oral Method* requires keeping the thermometer bulb in place in the pocket under your tongue with your mouth closed.
- The *Vaginal Method* requires placing the bulb about one inch into the vaginal canal as you lie on your back or side.
- The *Rectal Method* requires inserting the bulb into the rectal canal itself (not merely between the buttocks) as you lie on your stomach or side. Petroleum jelly on the bulb aids insertion.

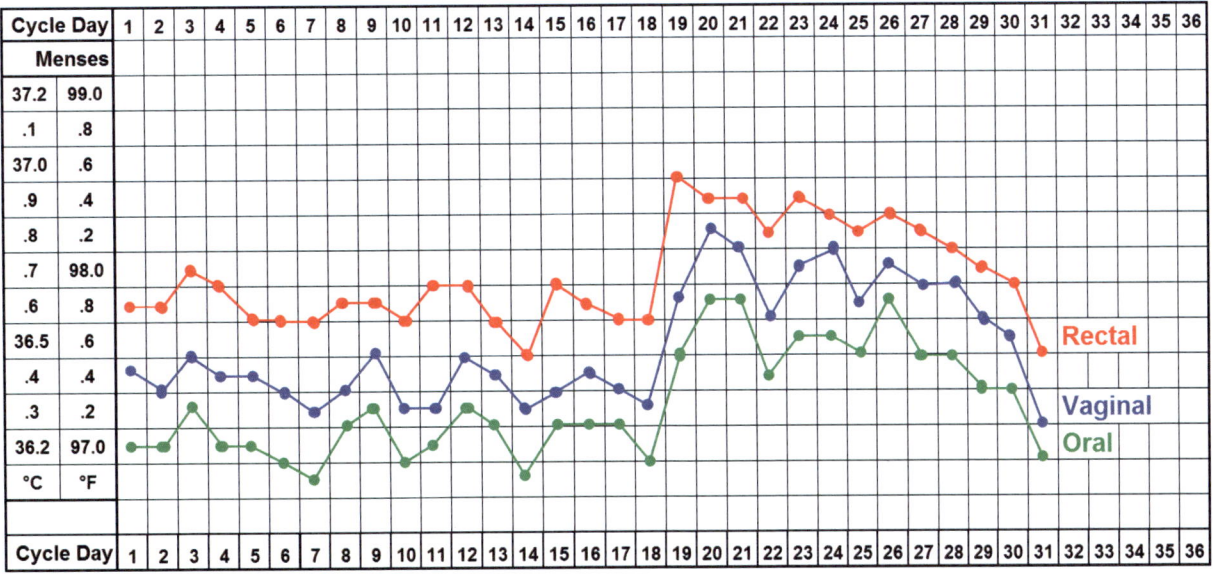

Stick with your chosen method of temperature taking for the entire cycle.

Don't switch from one method to another during the cycle. The readings won't be comparable. On any given day the oral reading is usually lowest and the rectal reading highest, with the vaginal reading in between.

If you have difficulty with one temperature-taking method, switch to another method at the start of the next cycle and note it on your chart. The oral method is sometimes a problem for women who have allergies and find it difficult to keep their mouth closed for that amount of time. Very few conditions affect the temperature of the vaginal or rectal canal, so either of these methods may give the easiest chart interpretation. Sometimes just taking the temperature a minute or two longer may help. Erratic temperature patterns are more often caused by poor temperature-taking technique and irregular schedules than by the thermometer itself. But make sure the thermometer is in good working order:

Spare Thermometer or Battery.

It is good to have an extra thermometer, or at least a spare battery, checked against the one in use so you will know if there is any difference in the temperature reading of the new one. Any slight temperature difference can be considered when interpreting your chart.

Consistency Is Essential

To obtain an accurate waking-temperature record useful for NFP, one must follow sound temperature-taking techniques. Consistency is the most important factor for getting a useful temperature record. To show only fertility-related changes on your chart, try to minimize other influences. This means it is best to take your temperature every day, under the same conditions, using the same method, immediately upon waking (before you rise, eat, drink, smoke, shower, exercise or do any physical activity). Some women take their temperature immediately after rising to care for a baby — this usually will not disturb the temperature. Others take their temperature daily while up and about doing routine light tasks right after waking. It is possible to get a usable record this way if the routine is consistent every day. Light activity rarely affects the temperature reading; however, "in bed upon waking" is preferable.

As mentioned, the human person has natural body rhythms (circadian rhythms) which fluctuate over a 24-hour time period. It is known that the basal body temperature is lowest in the early morning and highest in the afternoon. To have the clearest temperature pattern, take your temperature about the same time each day upon waking, even when you awaken earlier or later than usual. It is best to retire before midnight and to take your temperature before 7:30 a.m. or else note it on your chart. A variation of as much as ninety minutes from earliest to latest readings (forty-five minutes before or after the usual temperature taking time) should not disturb the accuracy of your temperature record, provided all the readings were taken before 7:30 a.m. If you vary from the usual conditions on a particular day, take your temperature anyway, and note the time on your chart. Read and record your temperature as soon as possible after taking it. Your digital thermometer should have the capacity to recall the last reading. If you are using a glass basal body temperature, the actual reading will be maintained until it is shaken down.

It takes 21 days to learn a new habit – Before you know it you'll be observing and charting without thinking about it!

Chart each day's reading in the column for that cycle day. Connect the dots as you go. But if you miss a day, just leave it blank — don't draw a connecting link across missed days. Note on your chart anything significant that might disturb the reading. It is possible to obtain a reliable temperature with only one to three hours of sleep, if it is taken at the usual time.

Some potential disturbances are: taking your temperature significantly later or earlier than usual (including spring and fall time changes), excessive alcohol consumption the night before, or illness, using a different thermometer, jet lag, altitude change, less than an hour of sleep just before waking, or unusual chill or heat (furnace out, changing the electric blanket temperature, children in bed). Fever spikes are easy to spot (you feel ill anyway). Medications don't, as a rule, affect the temperature.

What if you work evenings or on a rotating shift?

It is possible to get a clear temperature pattern if you wake up after 7:30 a.m. In such a case, the woman should take the reading at the same time each day (the earlier, the better).

For example, if Chelsea works from 3:00 p.m. to midnight, and wakes up at 9:00 a.m. each day, then she should try to consistently take her temperature at 9:00 a.m. Time variations after 7:30 a.m. usually are more significant, so Chelsea needs to be attentive to take her temperature at the same time every day.

Rene, on the other hand, works on a rotating shift. One week she works days, the next the night shift, and the third, she works graveyard shift. Rene needs to take her temperature when she wakes up, whatever time that may be. She should note the varying times down during the learning phase to see if her sleep pattern disturbs her temperature. If she has adjusted to this work pattern, it shouldn't pose a problem. If she notices an erratic temperature pattern, then more emphasis will need to be given to the cervical mucus and cervix signs.

Do you have to take your temperature every day?

It is good to take your temperature every day for one to two cycles to see the complete temperature pattern. You will learn, however, that only about nine or ten temperatures are essential. Cutting back comes only with experience.

Key Points:
- Consistency is important with temperature taking.
- Take your temperature daily either orally, vaginally, or rectally before 7:30 a.m.
- Note all disturbances.
- For instructions on variations to temperature taking methods read through this section again.

The Tissue-Paper Exam

It is not uncommon to hear women learning about cervical mucus say, "I thought I had an infection or something every cycle! It's so good to understand this discharge is normal." Women can learn to notice a cervical mucus discharge at the vaginal entrance during part of their cycle. This is a normal occurrence. Fertility is dependent upon the cervical mucus — it means that the woman's body is preparing for ovulation.

The onset of the cervical mucus flow is one of the indicators of the Possibly Fertile Time. In a typical cycle, the mucus is at first sticky and cloudy, then it progresses to a stretchy, clear, lubricative condition, much like raw egg-whites, before changing back to sticky mucus or dryness about the time of the temperature rise. There may be dry days after menstruation and during the established high-temperature phase.

You can monitor the cervical mucus sign during your daily personal care in as little as 30 seconds each check. To observe the cervical mucus pattern, follow a simple procedure known as the tissue-paper examination. Whenever you go to the bathroom to urinate (day or night), take white, unscented toilet tissue paper and fold it flat into a pad several layers thick. Some women experience an allergic response to colored or scented toilet tissue, so the recommendation is for white, unscented tissue. Then do what is referred to as the finger test. Here is the observation procedure:

- **WIPE** from front to back between the lips at the vaginal entrance while being attentive to whether or not the toilet tissue glides. Decide when wiping whether the tissue is gliding easily. It should be obvious to you at the time you wipe.

- **LOOK** at the folded toilet tissue to see whether there is any discharge on it or not and if there is...
- **TEST** what can be lifted off between the thumb and index finger to see how stretchy it is, whether it is clear or not, and what coloration it has, if any.

The tissue check should be done *before and after every voiding and bowel movement* because urination could wash away cervical mucus present beforehand, and because urination or a bowel movement could bring cervical mucus down. If no cervical mucus is observed during the day, this procedure should be done again, *before retiring*, after bearing down to bring any cervical mucus down. It is also prudent to check *during the night* if you get up to go to the bathroom.

To learn your pattern well, it is important to establish a *habit* of checking before and after, *every time*.

If you are *uncomfortable* with the finger test, *you may prefer to close and open* the toilet tissue to observe qualities of the cervical mucus. It is important to judge the qualities while stretching it either between the fingers or the toilet tissue.

To chart, you must decide at the end of the day if the day was:

1. **A TISSUE-DRY day** (charted Ø)

On a *Tissue-Dry Day*, the toilet tissue never glides and no cervical mucus is present. It may show nothing at all, or dampness from urine or perspiration, or "shine" from vaginal cells. Shine is a thin, clear film that can't be lifted off; it absorbs into the toilet tissue when rubbed lightly.

Shine is not considered "mucus." It is really vaginal fluid, and it doesn't have the "body" that cervical mucus does: it won't mound up on the tissue. If you finger-test shine, you'll find that it does not pull apart in threads.

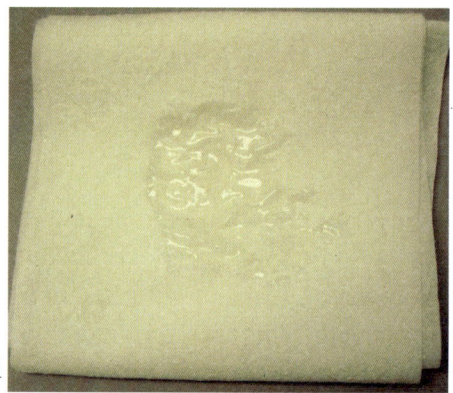

Dry -"Shine"

Chart Ø and call it a *Tissue-Dry Day,* if the tissue never glides and no mucus can be lifted off the tissue.

2.... or a **STICKY-MUCUS day** (charted **M**)

On a *Sticky Mucus Day*, mucus may be lifted off the tissue. The tissue never glides, the mucus never stretches an inch or more, and it is always "cloudy" throughout; that is, it's opaque, like wax paper, or even solid-colored.

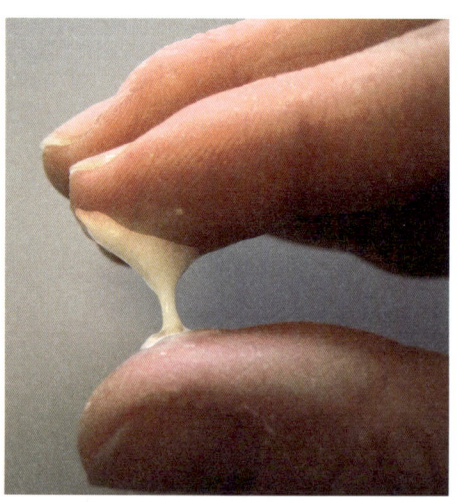

Sticky-Mucus

You chart **M** at the end of the day if this was the only kind of mucus you had and even if you saw it only once.

You also chart **M** for a "pasty" discharge, which mounds up, but just pulls apart; you cannot draw a pasty discharge into a thread. It is usually distinctly solid-colored, as opposed to being merely cloudy, and is similar to hand lotion or flour paste. While learning it is helpful to chart the traits below the observation.

> ### The Traits of **M** Can Be:
> ¼ = mucus stretches no more than ¼" before breaking.
> ½ = mucus stretches about ½" - ¾" before breaking.
> O = mucus is opaque like wax paper.
> P = pasty mucus, ¼", opaque, solid white or yellow without threads.

3.... or an **EGG-WHITE MUCUS day** (charted **EW-M**)

On an *Egg-White Mucus Day*, you will notice one or more of the following characteristics at least once or perhaps more often throughout the day:

The tissue-paper glides when you wipe it over the vaginal entrance or the mucus stretches an inch or more when you finger-test it or the mucus is "transparent"; that is, the mucus is clear like plastic wrap. The mucus is considered "transparent" even if only part of it is clear. You chart **EW-M** at the end of the day if even one of these characteristics occurred even once during the day.

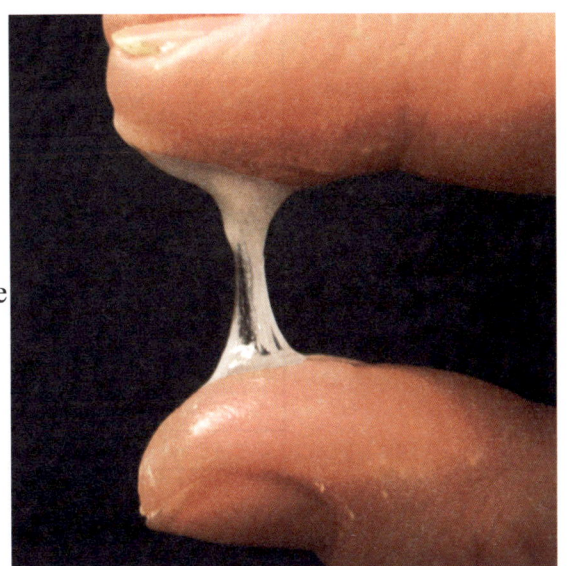

Egg-White Mucus

> ### The Traits of **EW-M** Can Be ...
> 1 = mucus stretches an inch or more.
> OT = mucus is mixed (part is opaque and part is transparent).
> T = mucus is transparent throughout like plastic wrap.
> G = tissue glides. Whenever the tissue glides, chart EW-M ... even if there seems to be no mucus to lift off.

Whenever the tissue-paper glides easily, chart EW-M...even if there seems to be no mucus to lift off.

Tissue glide means you are observing a highly fertile EW-M, a "hydrogel" that is more than 98 percent water. Glide is observed as a feeling of slippery-lubrication. Some women describe it as if "wiping with the tissue after intercourse" or feeling like "one needs to wipe with the tissue again." At the most fertile time, the cervical mucus can become so thin it is noticeable only by tissue glide or by a slippery- or runny-wet feeling at the vaginal entrance.

Charting Traits

#1 Cycle Day	1	2	3	4	5	6	7	8	9	10	11	12	13	14	15	16	17	18	19
Menses	■	■	■	■	■														
37.2 / 99.0																			
.1 / .8 Sensation																			
37.0 / .6											EW	EW	EW	EW	EW				
.9 / .4 Tissue							Ø	Ø	M	M	M	M	M	M	M	Ø	M	M	Ø	Ø
.8 / .2									P	¼"	1"	1"	1"	1"	G		¼"	¼"		
.7 / 98.0									O	OT	T	T	T			O	O		
.6 / .8											G	G	G						
36.5 / .6																			
.4 / .4																			
.3 / .2																			
36.2 / 97.0																			
°C / °F Cervix																			
Cycle Day	1	2	3	4	5	6	7	8	9	10	11	12	13	14	15	16	17	18	19

Charting Mucus Traits

- It helps to chart the traits of the cervical mucus as well as Ø, M, or EW-M symbols as displayed in the box above while you are learning.
- Charting Traits: An anxious new learner may overread the sensation of "glide." If you are noticing many "glide-only" days, even into the high-temperature phase, please make careful notations and discuss this with your NFP Provider.
- If a "stretchy" discharge continues into the high-temperature phase, please note the traits, and discuss this with your NFP Provider.
- You may find additional abbreviations for color helpful: e.g., "y" for yellow. Sometimes EW-M is tinged faint yellowish or pink, red, or brown, from a little blood in the mucus.
- Menstrual flow and other bleeding are charted as shown on page 33. All bleeding should be charted.

Making the Decisions

Throughout the day you observe and then at night you ask: "What was the most fertile sign I observed today?" Even if you only noticed it once during the day, that is all it takes! You only chart the day's most fertile sign and what you actually observed (not what you observed "most of the time" or what you might think you "should have" observed). Every woman has her own pattern and discovers it in due time.

Factors that disturb the cervical mucus.

There are a few things you need to be aware of when charting. Douching and vaginal sprays aren't really needed. Daily baths or showers are sufficient for hygiene purposes. The only exception is a prescribed douche. This treatment would need to be taken into account when interpreting the cervical mucus pattern.

It is the scenting agents in the items listed at right, including fabric softeners, that may irritate and disturb the natural cervical mucus process. Some women are more sensitive to such products than others and will be more apt to experience irritation. The unscented and milder forms of these products do not seem to pose a problem.

> **Avoid the Following ...**
> - Douching, vaginal sprays, bubble baths, and bath oils that are perfumed or irritating in any way.
> - Scented or colored toilet tissue, scented tampons or sanitary napkins, harsh detergents, and fabric softeners used in the clothes dryer with undergarments.
> - Undergarments made of synthetic fabrics unless there is a cotton crotch.
> - Tight slacks or jeans.
> - The IUD (intrauterine device), hormone drugs (especially the birth control pill, patches, injectables, implants, or cortisone), vaginal ring, and barrier contraceptives (condom, diaphragm, spermicides, or sponge).

Undergarments made of synthetic fabrics may make it hard to perceive the various vaginal sensations accurately. Cotton is recommended (it breathes easier and is less likely to lead to vaginal infections or irritation). It is best to avoid using tampons on light-flow days (use mini-pads instead). When tampons are used, they should be changed at least every four hours and not used while sleeping.

The IUD, the Pill, patches, injectables, and implants, and barrier contraceptives can make useful cervical mucus observations difficult or impossible.

Talcum-based powder warning: a study published in the *American Journal of Epidemiology* (March 1997) found a 50% increase in the risk of ovarian cancer for women using these products in the genital area.

Key Points:
- Follow the "Wipe, Look, Test" method to observe for cervical mucus every time you go to the bathroom, before and after each time you urinate or have a bowel movement.
- Fold the tissue flat and wipe from front to back in order to observe for gliding and to have the best mucus observation.
- Each day chart the most fertile sign: Ø, M, or EW-M along with the traits.

> **Be Sure to Chart ...**
> - Every day at the end of the day.
> - The most fertile sign of the day.
> - What you actually observed.
> - Note any possible disturbances.

The Vaginal Sensations

Some women have the feeling as if they're starting their menstrual period but think it is too early. When they go to check, there is nothing there. They were probably noticing vaginal sensations that occur within the vagina or at the lips of the vagina. This is another way to observe for the beginning of the fertile time. These vaginal sensations are perceived during the day. They are similar to other bodily sensations, such as the perception of a "dry" mouth, perspiration, or watery eyes. The vaginal sensations are experienced entirely apart from the tissue-paper exam. What you *feel* by sensation is as important as what you *see* by doing the tissue exam. There are three sensation observations listed from least fertile to most fertile:

1. **Sensation-Dry** (charted **d**): may be a positively dry, somewhat disagreeable, slightly itchy feeling, or a feeling of "nothing" *at the lips* of the vagina.

2. **Moistness** (charted ^m_M): a feeling from *within* the vagina of "something," as if "secreting moisture," or "shedding a tear *inside* the vagina," or "something flowing down inside the vagina," or "small bubbles bursting *inside* the vagina."

3. **Lubrication** (charted **L**): a feeling *at the lips* of the vagina of slipperiness, or a very distinctly runny-wet feeling *inside* the vagina—both are due to highly-fertile EW-M.

> **You Need To...**
> - Chart your tissue and sensation observations separately.
> - At the end of the day chart the most fertile sensation of the day.
> - The range from least to most fertile is d, ^m_M, L.

Always chart tissue and sensation separately. Attention to dryness and moistness is particularly important on the tissue-dry days after menstruation. *Lubrication* is important to notice toward the peak of the mucus episode.

Sometimes there is confusion between moistness and lubrication. *Moistness* is a "watery" feeling whereas lubrication is an "oily" one. The first noticeable change toward a more fertile sign is what tells you the fertile time is beginning.

> **For Purposes of Chart Interpretation:**
>
> **Sensation   Tissue**
> - d felt   =   Ø seen.
> - ^m_M felt   =   M seen.
> - L felt   =   EW-M seen.

Surprisingly, when you are attentive, you may be "Tissue-Dry but not Sensation-Dry," or "Sensation-Dry but not Tissue-Dry." When this happens, you assume fertility based on the more fertile sign of the two. This means that even if the day is Tissue-Dry (Ø), but you felt moistness or lubrication, you would correspondingly treat it as a Sticky-M or an EW-M day in applying the rules. It may take longer to recognize and chart confidently the range of sensations.

Generally, the changes in sensation mirror changes in the estrogen level and the fertile time. Sensation-Dry usually means a low estrogen level and lubrication indicates a high estrogen level. Even so, the ability to notice differences in sensation is something that varies from woman to woman and is the result of a gradual learning process.

It is also important to remember that no two women are exactly alike, and no two cycles in a given woman's life will be exactly alike. But you can notice things which are "typical" for you.

You need to learn your individual cervical mucus pattern: how the mucus usually starts, how rapidly it changes, and how long it lasts.

Key Points:
- Be attentive to vaginal sensations throughout the day.
- Chart the vaginal sensations separately from the toilet tissue observations.
- Each day chart the most fertile sign: d, $\frac{m}{M}$, or L.

Peak Day

To determine that you are again in the infertile time after a mucus episode, it is important to identify what is called the "Peak Day" (PK) Peak Day is a marker by which the infertile time will be measured. Peak Day is noticed in retrospect, and you will still be fertile for a few days afterwards. In other words, you won't be able to know a given day is Peak Day until a day or two later.

In a mucus episode, the Peak Day is the last day of the most fertile sign by tissue or sensation. Peak Day is the final day of any trait of EW-M or L, but if no EW-M or L is observed, it is the final day of any M or $\frac{m}{M}$. Note the following two examples:

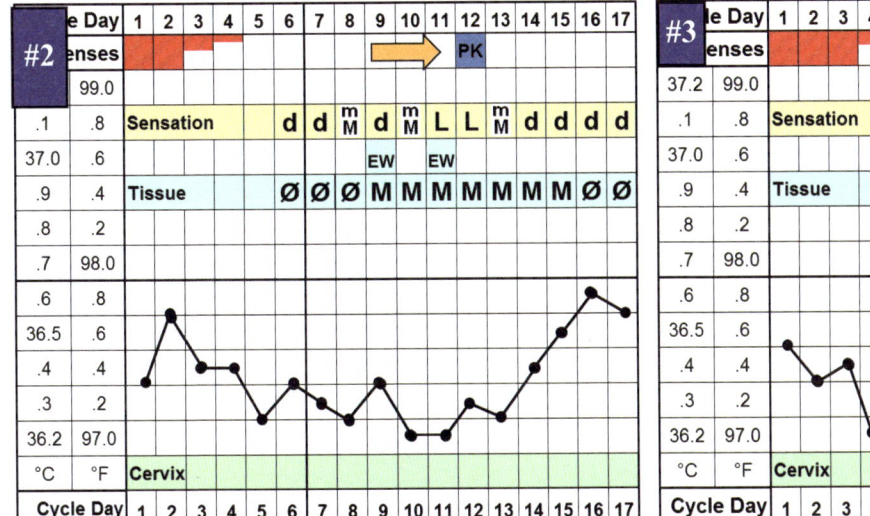
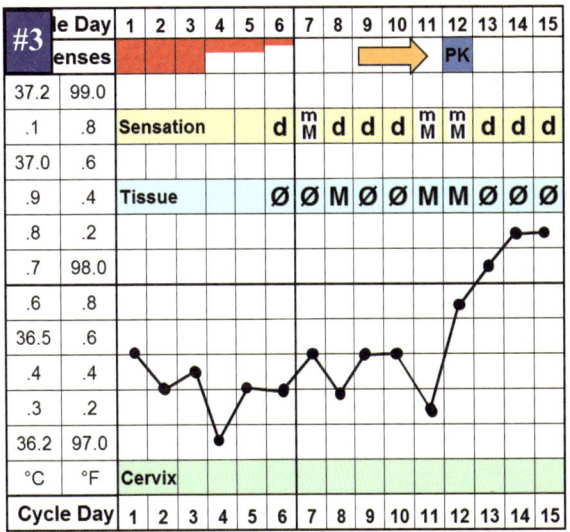

Sometimes lubrication or glide persists even after the mucus seems to have changed, diminished, or disappeared by tissue exam. Don't ignore this important observation. Toward Peak Day, the mucus may be more than 98 percent water, and thus, thin and clear. You may still have a lubricative sensation at the vaginal entrance but be unable to see or pick up any mucus. As long as there is any feeling of lubrication, you know you are not past the Peak Day. Intermenstrual bleeding (see page 32) is considered equivalent to EW-M and must be taken into account when establishing Peak Day.

The day of greatest amount of cervical mucus often occurs one or two days before Peak Day. Go by quality when setting Peak Day, not quantity.

Setting Peak Day correctly is important.

Peak Day is a reference point for applying the Sympto-Thermal Rule and the Basic Mucus Rule, two of the basic guidelines used in NFP.

Identifying Peak Day in a mucus episode is done separately from the temperature pattern. It is the last day of the best quality mucus sign observed in the mucus pattern. In certain situations, such as during stress or after childbirth, there can be more than one mucus episode before the temperature rise. In other words, it is possible to have more than one "Peak Day" per cycle. That doesn't mean, however, a woman ovulates more than once a cycle. It means she had fluctuating hormone levels with a changing mucus pattern in which ovulation did not result. A mucus pattern associated with ovulation will be followed by a sustained temperature rise.

> **Important Points to Remember about Peak Day:**
> - It is only known in retrospect, several days later, after observing the change from the best quality to a lesser quality mucus sign (even to dryness).
> - Peak Day is the final day of any trait of EW-M or L; but if no EW-M or L is observed, it is the final day of any M or ^m_M.

Peak Day was given its name because it is closely associated with the spiking "peak" of luteinizing hormone (LH) which surges just before ovulation. We cannot, however, pinpoint any day as being exactly the day ovulation occurs. Ovulation occurs within a few days before or after the Peak Day that is accompanied by a temperature rise. We can only be sure that a Peak Day is related to ovulation when a temperature rise follows.

If a temperature rise occurs along with the Peak Day, the post-ovulatory Completely Infertile Time can be applied utilizing the Sympto-Thermal Rule (see Chapter Three). If for some reason, there is a Peak Day and no temperature rise, you must continue to assume pre-ovulatory Relatively Infertile Time in accord with the Basic Mucus Rule (see Chapter Three). If you usually cycle on a monthly basis, it is possible stress is affecting your cycle. If you are discontinuing hormonal contraceptives, or are postpartum or premenopausal, or if you typically have cycles longer than 39 days, the Basic Mucus Rule may be a good choice. Check with your NFP Provider on the matter.

What if you are unable to observe any fertile signs by tissue or sensation? Peak Day must then be set by the signs at the cervix itself (see page 31).

Pinpointing the Range of Ovulation

The observation and charting techniques involved with NFP use cannot pinpoint the hour, or even the day, of ovulation. Ovulation detection can only be reliably done with ultra-sound or some laboratory techniques. It doesn't really matter, however, since the information that is observed and charted does clearly indicate the beginning and end of the woman's potentially fertile days. For example, the woman will experience several changes surrounding ovulation. She will notice a rise in her *basal body temperature* of about one-half of one degree Fahrenheit. Her *cervical os* or opening will become lower, closed, and firm. The cervical mucus in the cervical crypts will change, becoming thick, turning white or yellow, with little or no stretch to it. Externally, the woman typically notices a return to dryness.

The guidelines in this book consider the range of the fertile time. Ovulation may occur as early as three days before the cervical mucus Peak and up to three days afterward. The range of ovulation in relation to the cervical changes is similar. Ovulation can occur as early as the fourth last low temperature to as late as the second or third high temperature. These factors are considered when establishing effective guidelines for avoiding a pregnancy. Each sign contributes in its own way to the whole picture.

Key Points:
- Peak Day is the final day of any trait of EW-M or L, but if no EW-M or L is observed, it is the final day of any M or ^m_M.
- The day of greatest amount of cervical mucus often occurs one or two days before Peak Day. Go by quality when setting Peak Day, not quantity.
- Setting Peak Day correctly is important. It is a reference point for applying the Sympto-Thermal Rule and the Basic Mucus Rule, two of the basic guidelines used in NFP.

The Cervical Signs

Cervical mucus *originates* at the cervix, so it makes sense that this observation might be important to some women. The internal cervical exam involves observing the internal cervical mucus and the changes in the cervix. **While it is not necessary to observe the cervix many women find this particular observation very helpful.** There are four characteristics to be noted:

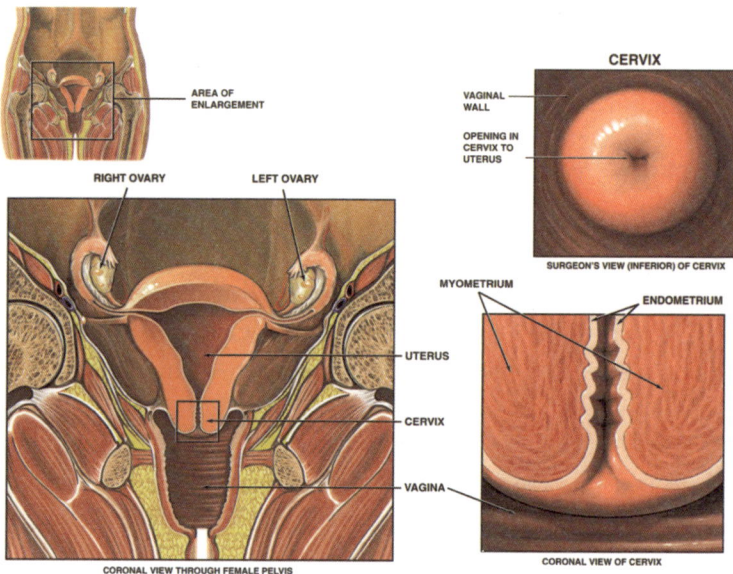

1. The degree of the *firmness* or *softness* of the cervix. Is it firm to the touch like the tip of the nose? Or is it soft like the inside of the cheek? Or is it somewhere in between?

2. The *position* of the cervix in the vaginal canal. It rises at the onset of the fertile time and lowers afterward. While fertile, the cervix may be so high within the vaginal canal some women will not be able to reach it. Some women also notice that their cervix will tilt towards the front or back at this time.

3. The degree of *closure* or *openness* of the cervix. The cervical os (opening) is similar to a dimple when it is closed, gradually opening around the time of ovulation, then closing tightly again around Peak Day. The birth process affects the cervix. Women who have not given birth vaginally will generally describe the cervical opening like a slight dimple. After a woman has had a vaginal childbirth, the cervical opening is elongated.

4. The *absence* or *presence* of cervical mucus. The vaginal canal is always moist, so one must distinguish between vaginal fluid and cervical mucus. Vaginal fluid does not have the same substance as cervical mucus and will disappear quickly. Vaginal fluid may be similar to a hand-lotion fluid or flour paste. Cervical mucus will pull apart in threads.

When observing the cervix, one relies on touch to determine the height and texture of the cervix. Then, the woman can look at any cervical mucus obtained and chart it as either M or EW-M.

Checking the Cervix

Place one foot on a low chair or stool while you stand on the other foot. Then insert two fingers into the vaginal canal and reach for the upper portion of the cervix. Place the fingers on opposite sides of the cervix and draw the

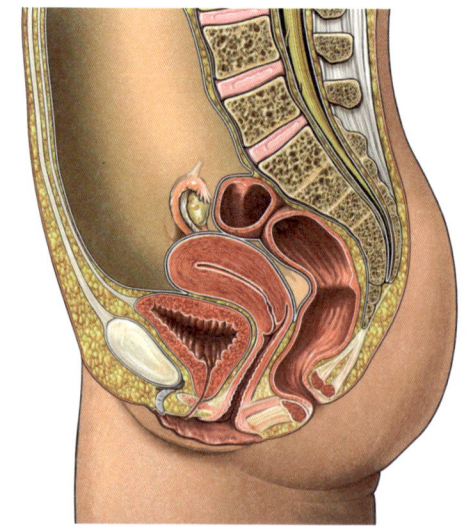

fingers downward while applying slight pressure on the cervix. If cervical mucus is present, it will gather between the fingers as they are drawn out. Then do the "finger-test" to check the mucus between the fingers, if any, for stretch, clarity, and amount. Since the vagina is a mucus membrane, there will be some mucus around the outside of the fingers as they are withdrawn. This fluid need not be considered for fertility purposes.

Some women find it easier to do this exam sitting or lying down or squatting (this is helpful if the uterus is tipped). When observing the cervix, you simply need to check the cervix at the end of the day after the last tissue-paper exam. To avoid concern over introducing an infection, you should have clean hands and trimmed nails. Women who have an active outbreak of vaginal herpes (HSV) or genital warts (HPV) should not check the cervix.

The Cervix Changes Throughout the Cycle

Some women do not notice all the indicators of the cervix, but find one or two helpful. For example, one woman will notice a dramatic change from high to low as the temperature begins to rise while another woman will instead notice the change from soft to firm. It generally takes several cycles of observing every day (except during menstruation) for the observations to make sense.

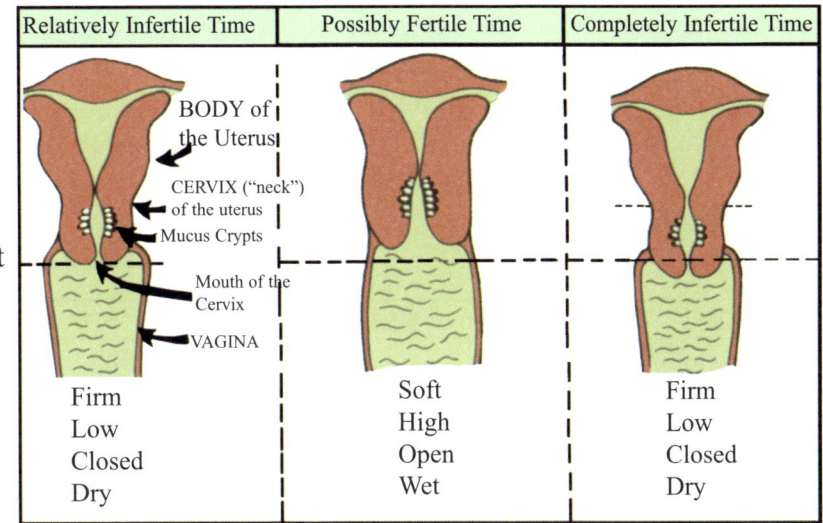

The key to confidence with the cervical check is to learn your pattern of change. For example, was the cervix today the same as yesterday? or relatively softer? or relatively firmer? The changes are usually relative and individual for each woman. The best way to learn the pattern is to observe the cervical signs and chart them daily. With your NFP Provider's help in evaluating your chart, use what information is relevant for you. Learn what is "firm" for you and what is "soft" for you, and so on. So be sure to chart the observations you make as best you can, even if you don't recognize a pattern at first.

Charting Cervix Observations

As long as the cervix remains unchanged after menstruation, you chart "F" and "C" for firm and closed. Chart "S" as soon as the cervix starts to become softer than before, and "O" as soon as it starts to become more open than before — in other words, when you notice a change. Keep on charting "S" and "O" until the cervix becomes firmer and more closed; then you chart "F" and "C" again. The same procedure can be used with "L" and "H" for low and high.

Some people like to chart the degree of opening and the level of the cervix as follows: they use a dot, small circle, and large circle for a closed, slightly open, and wide open cervix and place it lower or higher on the chart to indicate whether the cervix seems easier or harder to reach.

The observations for mucus at the cervix separately from the tissue:

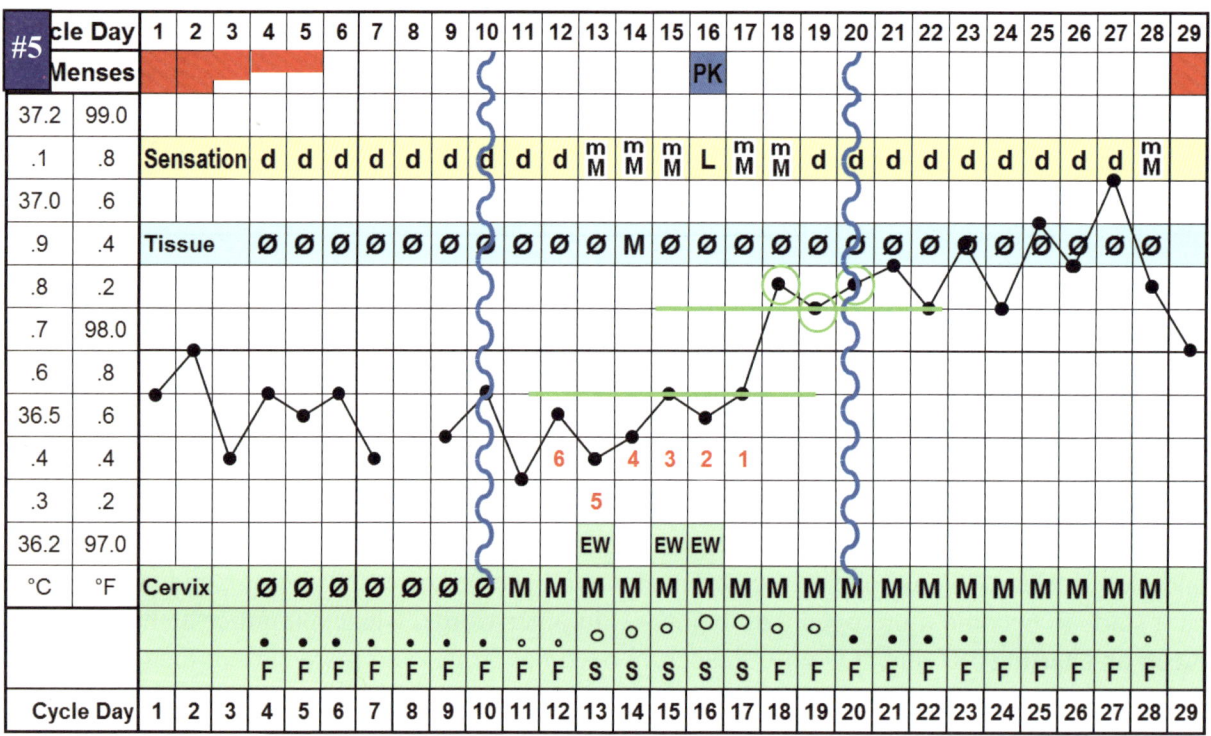

"**Cervix-dry**" (Ø) means no mucus is obtainable by compressing the cervix or else there is at most only a continuous thick yellow or white "discharge" (like hand lotion or flour paste) which is NOT cervical in origin (clarify this with your NFP Provider).

"**Cervix-wet**" (M or EW-M) means cervical mucus is now present, whereas before there was none. The mucus observed is charted M or EW-M according to the same criteria as the toilet tissue exam. It is distinguished from the cervix-dry observation because the discharge draws threads. During the fertile time cervical mucus typically "flows" from the cervix and bathes the vagina.

Charting the Cervix

Note: The vertical wavy lines block off the fertile time. Interpretation instructions will be covered in later chapters.

The best time to learn the cervix is to begin checking it right after menstruation or after the temperature has been high for several days. In both cases the cervix is usually firm, closed, and lower and easier to reach.

During menstruation the cervix may be slightly open. Immediately after menstruation it is usually firm and closed, unless this is a short cycle. Watch for the first noticeable change at the cervix. The first change may be from low to high, firm to soft, closed to open, or in the type of mucus observed.

Setting Peak Day by the Cervix. Peak Day is set by tissue and sensation, not by mucus noticed at the cervix. The only exception is when the woman is unable to notice any mucus symptoms by tissue or sensation. In such a case, the woman needs to rely on the cervix to set Peak Day.

Generally around the first day of high temperature, the cervix can be observed to change to a distinctly firm, low, and closed condition different from the way the cervix was firm, low, and closed after menstruation. Some couples appreciate this cervical sign because it confirms they will soon be in the Completely Infertile Time. This sign may also help to evaluate "Peak Day + temperature rise associated with stress/illness."

Charting the cervix signs can also help the woman be more certain about how to interpret the discharge after intercourse during the pre-ovulatory time.

The experience of Northwest Family Services is that one quarter of the women chart the cervix. The cervical exam can be of particular help to women who have a continuous discharge or a short episode of cervical mucus. For instance, if the cervix remains consistently firm, low, closed, and "dry" after menstruation, despite the presence of continuous discharge externally, there is assurance of infertility.

Key Points:
- Check the cervix at the end of the day in either a sitting, standing, lying down, or squatting position.
- Chart the FLCØ or SHOW (or M) or EW-M Signs.
- Only if there is no discernible Peak Day by tissue or sensation, is Peak Day set by the cervical mucus at the cervix or if you have questions contact your NFP Provider.

The Secondary Signs

The temperature, cervical mucus, sensation, and cervix are the "primary" signs and there are scientifically-based rules that effectively determine the fertile and infertile times. There are also "secondary signs" associated with the fertile and infertile times, but their occurrence is not consistent or accurate enough to develop rules. It is good, however, to understand and chart them. For instance, when a woman says, "I must be ovulating. I can feel it," she may be referring to intermenstrual pain. She may be noticing intermenstrual pain, but certain distinctions must be kept in mind to avoid confusion over jumping to conclusions regarding the day of ovulation.

1. Intermenstrual Pain (charted IP)

Intermenstrual pain (IP) relates to activity around the ovaries near the time of ovulation. One school of thought attributes the "pain" to the action of the fallopian tube as it rises up to the ovary around ovulation (Vollman). Yet another claims the swelling follicle as well as the process of the egg cell bursting forth yields the "pain" (Doyle, Hilgers). In any event, what is charted "IP" is felt as a sharp pain or as a crampiness, somewhat like the onset of menstrual cramps or dull lower back pain. IP is usually noticed only for a few hours and rarely for more than two days. IP as defined here occurs close to Peak Day and seems to be associated with elevated estrogen levels. It is incorrect to say IP pinpoints the day of ovulation. IP is not to be confused with menstrual cramps.

2. Breast Tenderness (charted BT)

Breast tenderness (BT) may begin with a prickly, tingling sensation, sometimes a sharp pain, in the breasts, more toward the nipples around Peak Day. Some women describe BT as "having sore nipples." This may change into a heaviness deeper in the breast tissue and be experienced as breast "tension" or "fullness" and finally as tender "lumpiness" just before menstruation. Breast tenderness reflects rising and elevated progesterone levels. In other words, BT is associated with the time after ovulation. This makes the Relatively Infertile Time the best time to do a monthly breast examination.

3. Intermenstrual Bleeding (charted [15|16])

Intermenstrual Bleeding may be noticed around Peak day. This bleeding may appear as red, brown, pink, or yellowish strands in the mucus or as full bleeding around the time of ovulation. A sudden drop in estrogen is the reason for its occurrence. This is not menstrual bleeding and is always considered fertile. Peak Day is set accordingly.

Key Point:
- Secondary signs are not consistent or accurate enough to develop rules, but it is helpful to understand and chart them.
- When using STM it is important to consistently chart the temperature and one other primary sign such as the tissue paper examination. As you gain the confidence in observing and charting, and which rules apply to your circumstances discuss with your NFP provider which signs make most sense for you right now.

How much time does it take to monitor your natural fertility?

- 2 minutes BBT
- 30 seconds per tissue paper check
- Mental note for sensation
- A moment to chart

Isn't self knowledge and your health worth it?

Charting All the Signs

Josh and Sarah Cummins have been charting for several years. She began menstruating at age 14 and was 29 at the time of her chart shown below. Her *gynecological* age, 15 years, is the number of years since her first menstrual period (menarche). She has 2 sons (M), no daughters (F), and has had 1 miscarriage (MC). She takes her daily temperature orally at 6:45 a.m. Josh charts the information Sarah observes during the day. At the beginning of each cycle, he takes a moment to mark the month, year, and date of the cycle days in advance on each new chart.

Out of the 38 cycles the Cummins have charted, Sarah's shortest recorded cycle is 27 days and her longest is 36 days. Her cycle range is then 27-36 days. A variation of a week or so between the shortest and longest cycle is considered typical.

This is cycle number 38 and it is a 29-day cycle. It starts with Day 1 of menstruation on February 17th and continues through March 17th, the last day before the new menstrual period. So Josh encircles Day 29 at the bottom of the chart to show it is the last day of the cycle.

Cycle Day 30, which is March 18th, is actually Day 1 of her next cycle. Josh will *start a new chart* with the first day of true menstruation, March 18th, as Day 1 on the new chart. Sometimes a woman is not sure which day menstruation began. For charting purposes, Day 1 = the first day of bright red flow. Premenstrual spotting is part of the previous cycle (See Day 29).

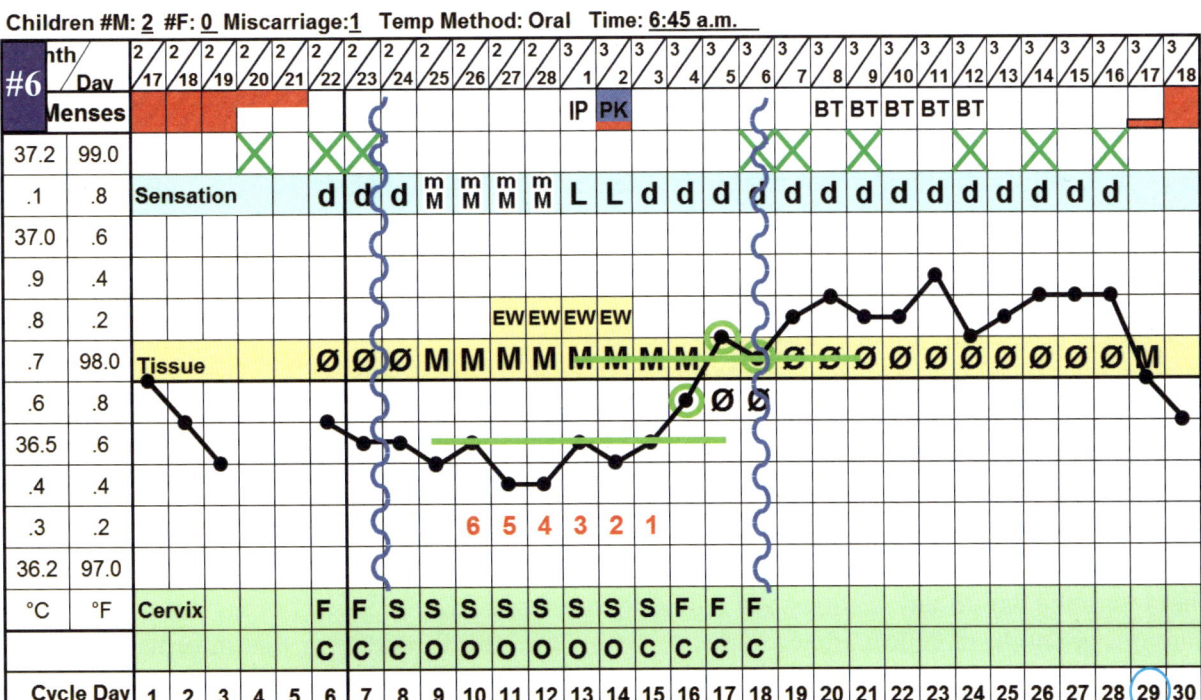

Tissue: Ø = Dry. M = Sticky Mucus. EW-M = Egg-White Mucus.

Sensation: d = Sensation-dry. $\genfrac{}{}{0pt}{}{m}{M}$ = Moistness felt. L = Lubrication felt.

Peak Day (charted "PK") is set by crosschecking tissue and sensation in almost all cases.

Cervix: F = firm, C = closed, S = soft, O = open. Josh starts charting S/O as soon as Sarah notices the cervix begin to soften/open. H and L = higher/lower. When compressing the cervix, cervix-dry (Ø) and cervix-wet (M or EW-M) are charted on the cervix line immediately above the F/L/C or S/H/O symbols.

Temperature: Taken upon waking. Note that dots are not to be connected across missed days (see Days 4 and 5).

Menstruation is heavy on Days 1-3, then light on Days 4-5. **Intermenstrual Pain** (IP) is on Day 13, **Intermenstrual Bleeding** (⬚) is on Day 14, and **Breast Tenderness** (BT) from Day 20 onward.

The **wavy vertical lines** are the way to mark the beginning and end of the fertile time. In this cycle, Day 7 was the last infertile day because a change was noticed at the cervix on Day 8. The fertile time lasted until evening on Day 18, when the Sympto-Thermal Rule was met (see Chapter Three). The record of intercourse and genital contact is complete.

Full intercourse is charted with the symbol "X." Any other **Genital Contact** is charted "GC." The last intercourse before the fertile time and the first intercourse after the fertile time, as well as any intercourse or genital contact during the fertile time, should be recorded. Any use of contraceptives should also be indicated — this is a matter of honesty, to determine the cause of pregnancy if it occurs, and to evaluate the mucus pattern.

Periodic abstinence is how pregnancy is prevented with NFP. For couples serious about avoiding a pregnancy, a more conservative approach is necessary at first. Josh and Sarah applied the 6-Day Rule and the Sympto-Thermal Rule for the first 6 cycles. Then they extended the Relatively Infertile Time by following the Early Dry Days Rule (see page 45 for rule) along with the Sympto-Thermal Rule for the Completely Infertile Time. For example, in Cycle 38 Chart #6 above, they abstained from Day 8 until evening of Day 18. At first the periodic abstinence was especially challenging. Then Josh and Sarah found other couples who also used NFP and they found that discussing its benefits and laughing about its challenges has helped them with the day-to-day realities. An online listserve provided support, but they're a bit cautious about the technical advice and stick with their NFP Provider for that information. Josh is pleased that the sacrifice means Sarah doesn't need to use artificial hormones. Sarah is proud of Josh's sacrifice. They are both finding a spark in their relationship which they haven't experienced for awhile.

CHAPTER THREE: NFP GUIDELINES

Observing and charting is important for gathering data about your fertility. This section begins with the easiest and most effective guidelines. Many couples are interested in the bottom line: "When am I (or she) infertile?"

For successful use of Natural Family Planning one needs to correctly interpret the chart and work with your NFP Provider to identify which rules fit your type of cycles. We'll begin by identifying the guidelines for the Completely Infertile Time (CIT) of the cycle. These rules depend on a sustained temperature rise which verifies that ovulation has occurred. The best approach to identifying CIT infertility is to follow a combination temperature-plus-cervical-mucus rule known as the Sympto-Thermal Rule.

The Basic Sympto-Thermal Rule

The Sympto-Thermal Rule (STR) identifies the Completely Infertile Time (CIT) — the infertile days after ovulation — in virtually all fertile cycles. The STR can easily be applied to a "biphasic" chart (one with a sustained temperature rise) provided the couple takes care to chart cervical mucus and temperature observations. It is a highly effective rule. Dr. Josef Roetzer's research shows a 99.9+ percent effectiveness rate from this rule. In order to achieve such high effectiveness a few simple steps are required. You will want to make a habit of following these steps and chart each cycle. Don't rely on estimating the interpretation by sight. The STR isn't like horseshoes — "close enough" just doesn't work. No woman is ever just "a little pregnant."

- To apply the S-T Rule there are several steps:
1. **Determine Peak Day (PK).**

Peak Day is usually the last day of any trait of EW-M or L. But if no EW-M or L can be observed, Peak Day is the last day of any M or $\genfrac{}{}{0pt}{}{m}{M}$. Peak Day involves crosschecking tissue and sensation. (If you see a temperature rise, but cannot determine Peak Day or if you are uncertain about this essential interpretation, call your NFP Provider for assistance.)

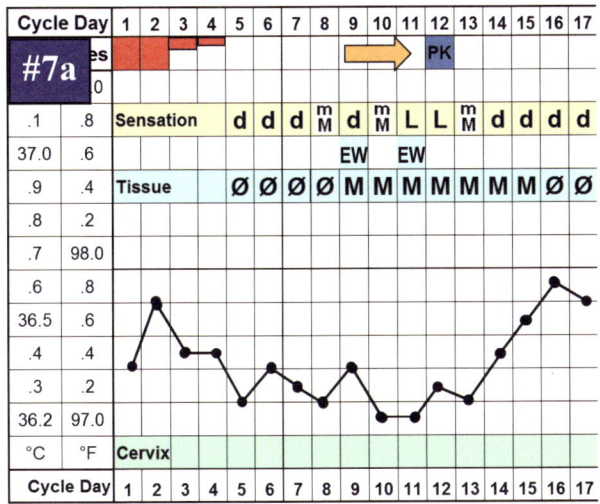
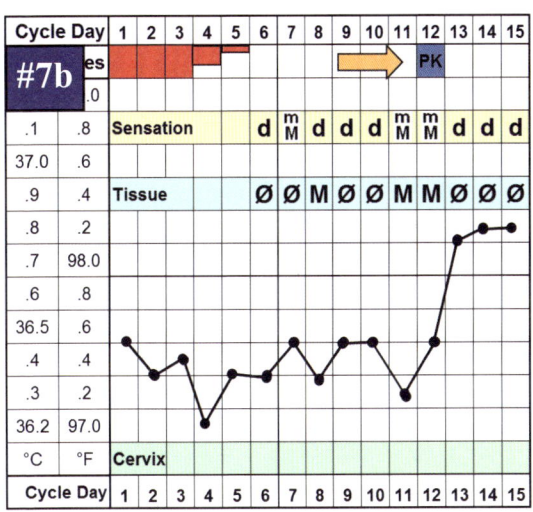

2. **Set the Pre-Rise Baseline (PRB).**

In order to evaluate your temperature rise, you need to be able to separate the high temperatures from the low temperatures. This is done by establishing what is known as the Pre-Rise Baseline or PRB. You can only set the PRB after you identify three days of undisturbed temperatures that are all higher than the six temperatures before the group of three highs. In other words, you need THREE higher than SIX. You will then reverse number the six low temperatures as seen in the example. The PRB is set by drawing a line through the HIGHEST undisturbed temperature of the final 6 low temperatures. **Any temperature above the PRB is considered a high temperature.**

A few important considerations.

- The temperatures can begin to rise around Peak Day, so you might see a temperature rise a day or two before or after Peak Day. The six last lows and the PRB are based on the temperature pattern and not on the location of Peak Day.
- Only the six last lows are considered when establishing the PRB. Higher temperatures earlier in the cycle are not used in setting the PRB.
- Generally, your PRB is fairly consistent from cycle to cycle. The PRB is usually within 0.1°F or 0.2°F of your usual pattern. If you have a PRB that is unusually low for you in a given cycle, especially if it is occurring earlier than usual, ask yourself if it might be affected by other factors. Call your NFP Provider before you apply the STR in such a case.
- Even though the PRB is similar each cycle, you need to draw it on your chart every cycle such as seen in the chart above.

3. Draw a second line, called a "**Full Thermal Shift Level**," (**FTSL**) line 0.4° F above the Pre-Rise Baseline. Note: if you are using Celsius, the FTSL is at 0.2° C above the Pre-Rise Baseline. The FTSL will assist you in knowing when you are infertile (e.g., the STR is fulfilled).

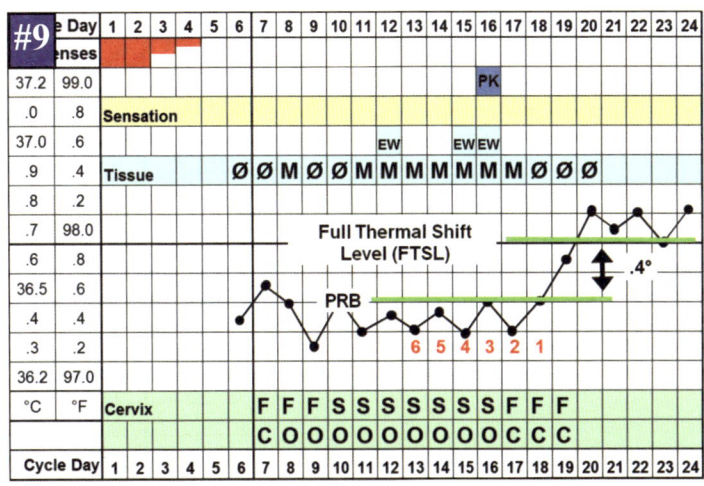

There can be many temperature patterns. Two of the most common temperature patterns are a rapid rise and a shallow rise. When there is a rapid rise in the temperature pattern, the STR is often fulfilled earlier than it would be with a shallower or slower temperature rise. The FTSL allows you to interpret your chart correctly.

4. **Encircle high readings that occur AFTER Peak Day**. Only very particular temperatures are encircled. Encircling temperatures is the way high temperatures AFTER Peak Day are noted. A "high" temperature means one that is "above the Pre-Rise Baseline." For example, the "high" temperature on Day 14 is not encircled because it is on Peak Day. Note that wavy lines denote onset of infertility.

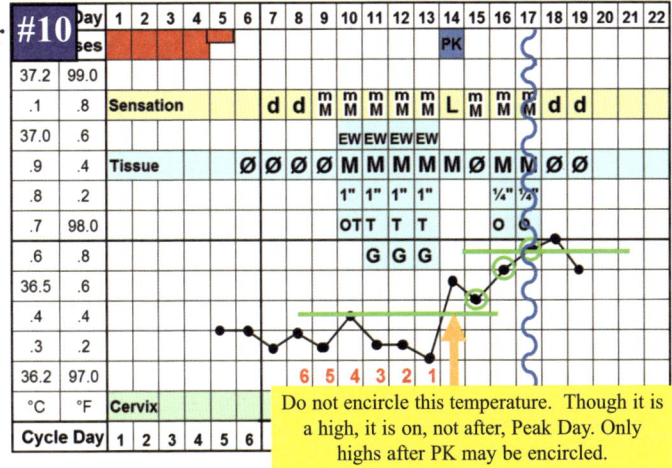

Encircled temperatures are like the countdown toward the infertile time. There are only three to five encircled readings. Once the STR is fulfilled, there is no need to encircle further temperatures. If a post-Peak temperature is not above the PRB, don't encircle it. If there are any high temperatures on or before Peak Day, don't encircle these temperatures. They are not part of the last six lows either.

5. **If the THIRD encircled reading is on or above the Full Thermal Shift Level line**, then the STR is met and the Completely Infertile Time starts that evening. The STR is fulfilled evening of Day 22 in this chart. Day 19 is not encircled because it is not high, even though it is after Peak Day. Note: Strictly speaking, the third encircled reading after Peak Day only needs to be "just about 0.4°F" above the PRB to assume the Completely Infertile Time that evening. "Just about 0.4°F or more" means 0.36°F or more (0.36°F = 0.2°C).

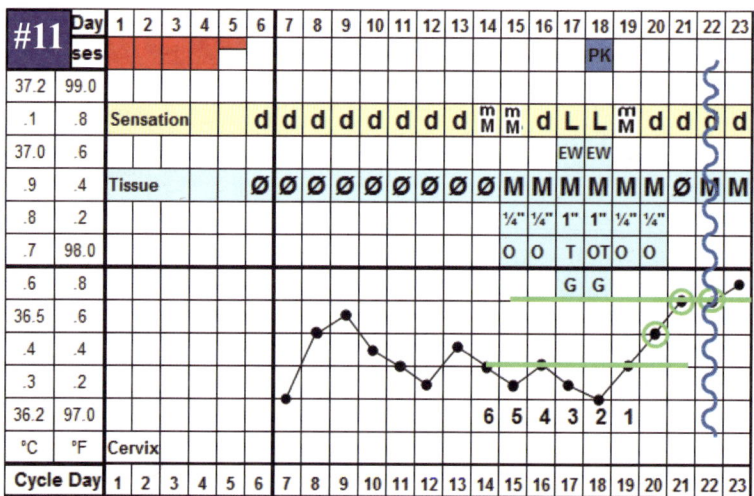

6. **If the third encircled reading is NOT on or above the Full Thermal Shift Level line, wait until evening on the FOURTH** encircled high reading before assuming the Completely Infertile Time. The fourth encircled high temperature need only be above the Pre-Rise Baseline. In fact, with four encircled temperatures, none of the temperatures need to reach the FTSL. Such a temperature rise is considered a shallow temperature rise.

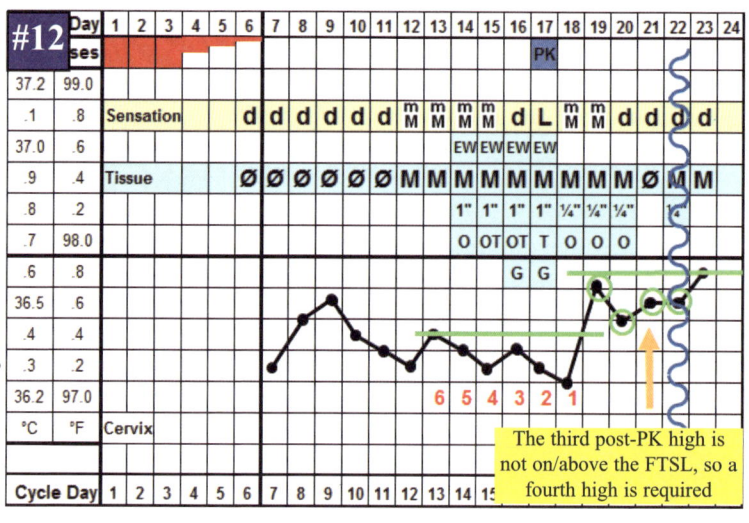

7. What if you had a fever during the six low temperatures or otherwise had **a disturbed temperature**? You can ignore an explained disturbance when setting the final six low temperatures. Put parentheses around disturbed temperatures.

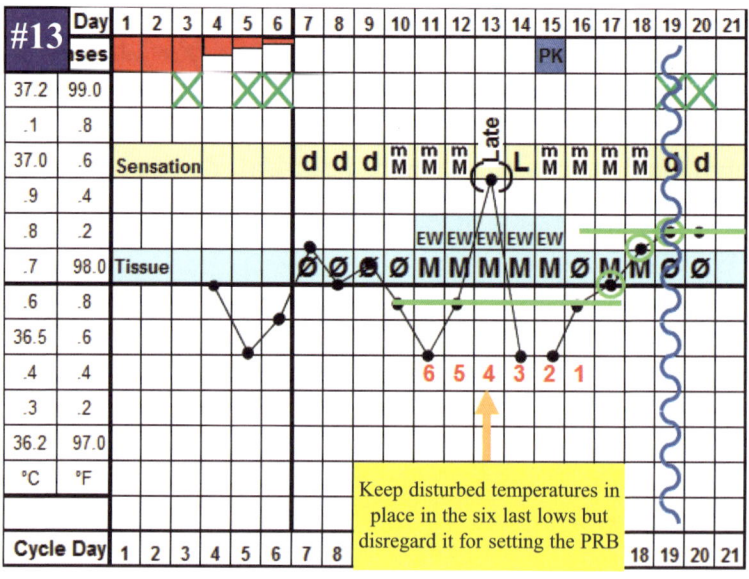

38

If some temperatures are missing or disturbed, don't extend the 6 low temperatures further back. Include the missing or disturbed temperatures as part of your six low temperatures, but do not use disturbed temperatures to set the PRB or FTSL. Day 13 in Chart #13 (on the previous page) is considered part of the 6 lows, but it is not considered when establishing the PRB. You need to have at least five undisturbed low temperatures to apply the STR. If you have more disturbed or missing temperatures in a given cycle, please refer to page 56, for information on the Mean Temperature Rule or to page 53, for information on the Basic Mucus Rule.

8. If after Peak Day there are at first one or two readings higher than the preceding six, then a one-day drop (See Day 15 on Chart 14) and a rise again, what do you do? **This is known as a one-day post-Peak drop.** If this pattern occurs, interpret your chart in the following way. Encircle three high temperatures after Peak Day. Apply the required encircled readings as previously described. On Chart #14, Day 17 is the third encircled reading and is 0.4°F above the PRB. The one-day drop is treated as a disturbed temperature and ignored in the interpretation.

9. **What if there is a "delayed temperature rise" after Peak Day?** In such a case, the STR assumes infertility the evening of Peak+5 with two high-temperature readings. These two encircled high temperatures only need to be above the PRB. This is known as a delayed, shallow temperature rise. In chart 15, Day 21 is Peak + 5 and is the evening of the second encircled reading. The infertile time begins in the evening. Both requirements must be fulfilled.

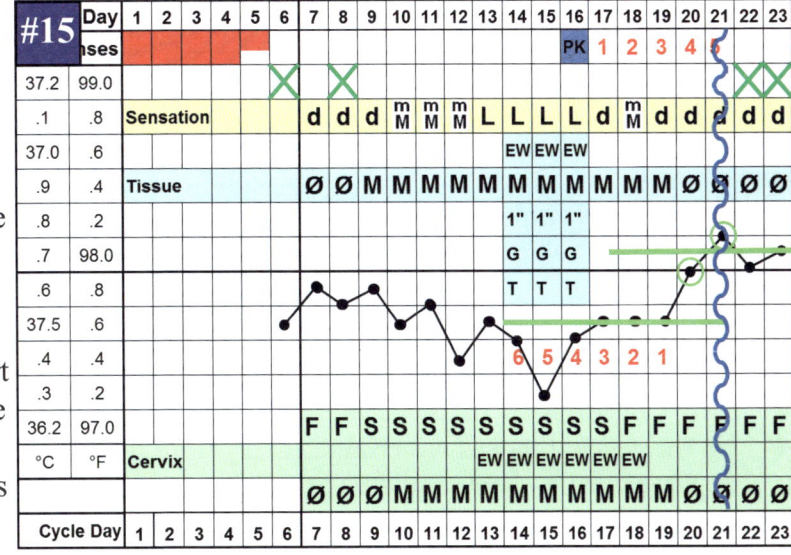

If your cervix usually changes to a distinctly firm and closed condition around the time of the temperature rise, three days of this distinctly firm, closed cervix confirms the "Peak+5 and 2 highs" as sufficient to assume infertility. Without the cervical check, it is prudent to continue to observe for cervical mucus and chart your temperature until a third or fourth higher temperature fulfilling the STR interpretation is charted.

10. What about the effects of **stress, illness, or traveling** that may occur around the time of mucus drying up + a temperature rise? Assume Completely Infertile Time when you are confident you have the necessary undisturbed high temperatures after Peak Day to fulfill the STR as described above. These temperatures should be at your usual high temperature level. Three days of a distinctly firm, closed cervix confirms the temperature interpretation.

11. **Post-Peak Stretch.** After a distinct temperature rise, some women observe a discharge that is opaque with no glide sensation; however, it can be pulled it apart 1" or more. Technically, this observation is considered EW-M. This condition is known as Post-Peak Stretch, and there is a special application of the STR if you notice this change in cervical mucus. You may reset Peak Day if the following conditions are met:

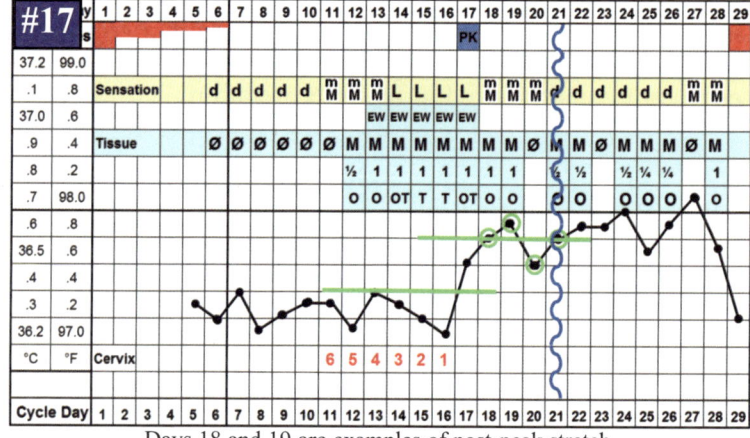
Days 18 and 19 are examples of post-peak stretch.

- There is an undisturbed, distinct temperature rise.
- No lubricative sensation is present.
- The cervical mucus has changed away from the EW-M qualities of gliding and clear. For example, there should be no clear strands of cervical mucus observed. The only remaining quality of EW-M is that it will stretch 1" or more. Stretch is the least important characteristic of EW-M. Sometimes the discharge can be stretched an 1" or more just because of the amount of cervical mucus present.
- When you observe a distinct change in the cervical mucus, even though the discharge stretches an 1" or more, reset Peak Day to the last day you observed EW-M with traits of transparent or glide, or you experienced a lubricative sensation.

- Chart the post-Peak stretch as "M" with a notation of 1" below it. (See Days 18-19 in Chart #17)
- This guideline can only be applied with an undisturbed temperature rise.
- You should identify this as a consistent pattern in at least two cycles before applying this adaptation to the third and subsequent cycles.

12. The Completely Infertile Time lasts until the end of the cycle. Couples for whom avoidance of pregnancy is of the highest priority should restrict intercourse to the Completely Infertile Time.

Key Points:
- The STR requires three high temperatures after Peak Day with the third temperature at 0.4°F or more above the PRB. There are variations to this rule for a shallow temperature rise or a delay in the temperature rise.
- If EW-M persists into the high-temperature phase, review the guidelines for post-Peak stretch above.

Relatively Infertile Time Rules

When a new cycle begins, new rules apply. The postovulatory Completely Infertile Time (CIT) lasts until the first day of menstruation, when the pre-ovulatory Relatively Infertile Time (RIT) of the new cycle begins. The RIT usually lasts at least six days, although the process leading up to ovulation can be quite variable in length.

The first day of "bright red flow" of true menstruation is the first day of a new cycle, so be sure to start a new chart with that day as Day 1.

It's best while learning NFP to take a more conservative approach such as following the 6-5-0 Day Rule described below. Beginners should gradually extend their use of infertile days during the RIT. Inexperienced couples who extend intercourse beyond the limits of the infertile time will likely become pregnant. Experience with cervical mucus, sensation, and cervix charting helps couples effectively use NFP. Work with your NFP Provider to determine which rules make the best sense for your use of NFP.

> Most couples in Typical cycles apply the Sympto-Thermal Rule and 6/5 Day Rule for the first 4-6 cycles. It is important for your success with NFP to work with your NFP Provider to decide which rule(s) make the most sense for you and your current circumstances.

The First Six Days: the 6-5-0 Day Rule

The first six days of a new menstrual cycle can be assumed infertile until midnight at the end of Day 6 with some qualifications. Which of the following is true for you?

[___] My **shortest cycle** was **26 days long or longer**. Assume Days 1-6 infertile.

[___] My **shortest cycle** was **23-25 days long**. Assume only Days 1-5 infertile.

[___] My **shortest** cycle was **22 days or less**. Assume 0 days infertile for now.

6-5-0 Day Rule	
Shortest Past Cycle	Assume Infertile
26 days or longer	6 days
23-25 days	5 days
22 days or less	0 days (for now)

The 6-5-0 Day Rule presupposes you have a sustained temperature rise before menstruation so you can identify *true menstruation*. In other words, you were able to apply the Sympto-Thermal Rule or some other temperature rule before you experienced your menstrual period.

6-5-0 Day Rule Chart

Chart #18 illustrates that the Sympto-Thermal Rule has been fulfilled. The woman has cycle lengths which are 26 days or longer, so the 6-Day Rule can be applied. That means that Days 1 through midnight of Day 6 are considered infertile. On the light flow days, the woman begins observing her signs to make sure there are no unexpected mucus observations. After Day 6, she assumes herself fertile again until the Sympto-Thermal Rule has been fulfilled. Women with typical cycles should follow this approach for 4 to 6 cycles before assuming Relatively Infertile Time rules beyond Day 6.

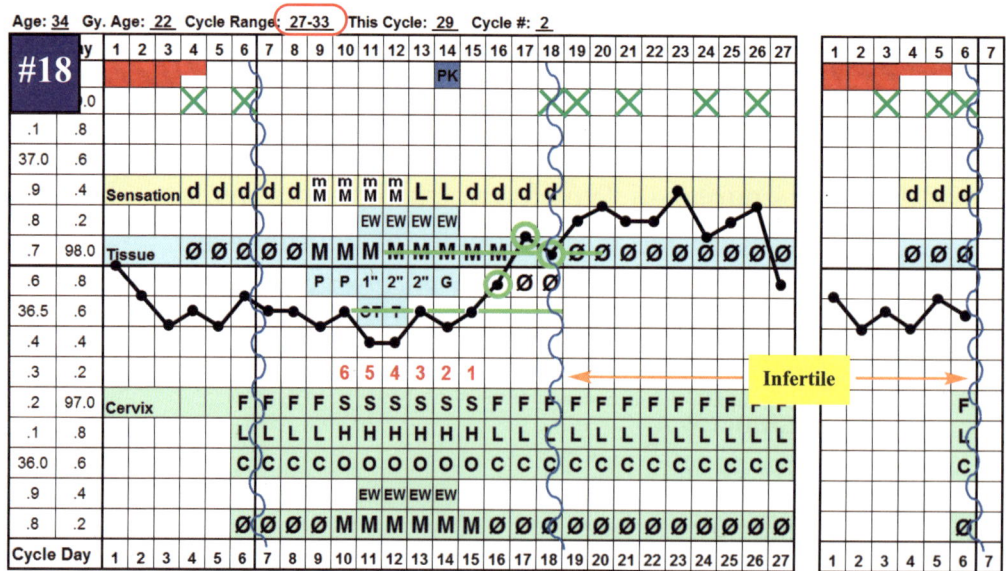

Some people think all bleeding can be treated as menstrual bleeding. This is NOT true. Only bleeding preceded by a high-temperature phase can be considered for the 6-5-0 Day Rule. Mid-cycle bleeding, such as seen on Days 24-26 in Chart #19, is considered fertile, even if it seems "just like menstruation." Any type of non-menstrual bleeding is treated as fertile; it could be masking cervical mucus and be associated with ovulation.

New Learner Cycle 2

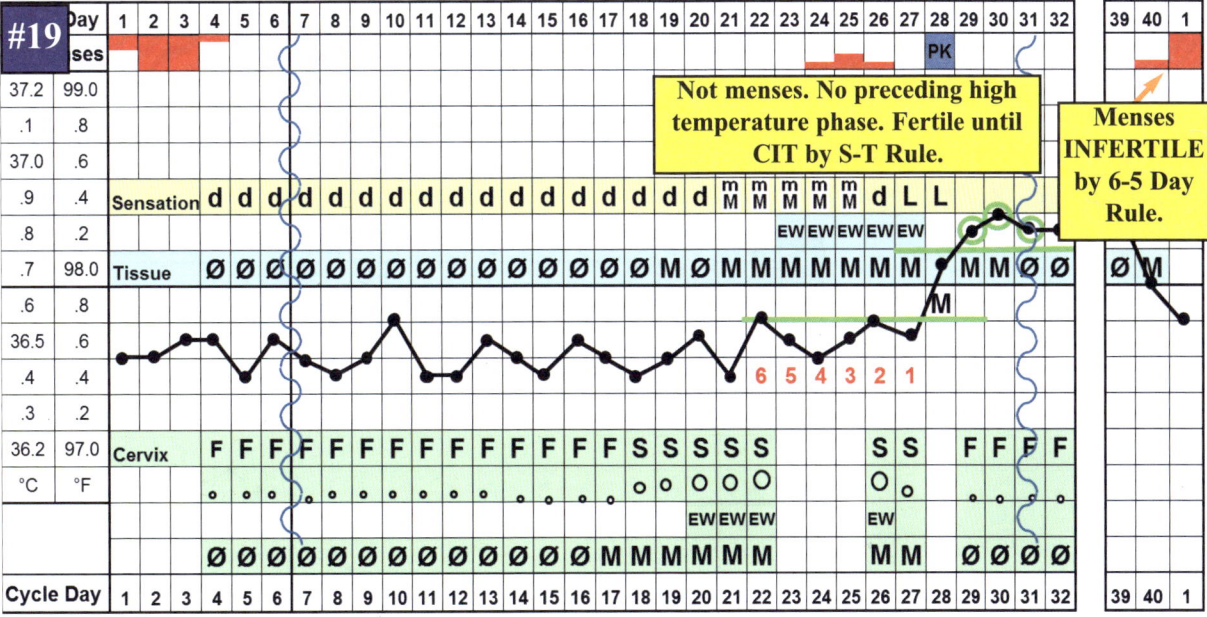

Bleeding Other than True Menses Is Fertile

Menstrual flow beyond Day 6 is considered fertile. It is the first five or six days that are assumed infertile, not menstrual flow as such; don't assume you are still infertile once beyond Day 6, just because there is still bleeding (see chart #20). For example, Days 7 and 8 in Chart #20 are considered fertile even though the menstrual flow has continued.

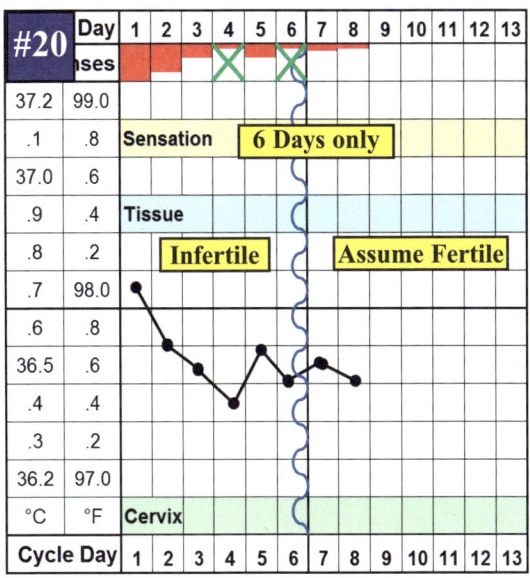

What about "mucus" on or before Day 6? If you have what seems to be EW-M on, say, Day 6, but aren't sure if it's cervical mucus, seminal fluid, or menstruation, you need to consider it fertile. If you don't usually have this EW-M early in your cycle, assume you may be having a short cycle, and abstain if avoiding pregnancy. Checking the cervix for a firm, closed cervix suggests infertility, however. Discuss any early EW-M with your NFP Provider.

The key to evaluating the significance of "short" cycles is *where the final 6 low temperatures lie.* Is the cycle short because of early ovulation and early fertility? or because of a short high-temperature phase? The temperature pattern will tell. If the final 6 lows are always later than Day 6 in your *shortest* cycles, you can still assume the first 6 days infertile (observe this for 4 to 6 cycles and discuss it with your NFP Provider; see also page 46 for more information on the significance of the final 6 lows for interpreting the mucus pattern).

For example, Chart 21 is a 22 day cycle from a woman who has a cycle range of 22-29 days. After consulting with the couple's NFP Provider and charting for 6 cycles, it was noted that the 6th last low temperature (see Day 8) never occurred earlier than Day 7. With this information it was determined the couple could continue to apply the 6-Day Rule.

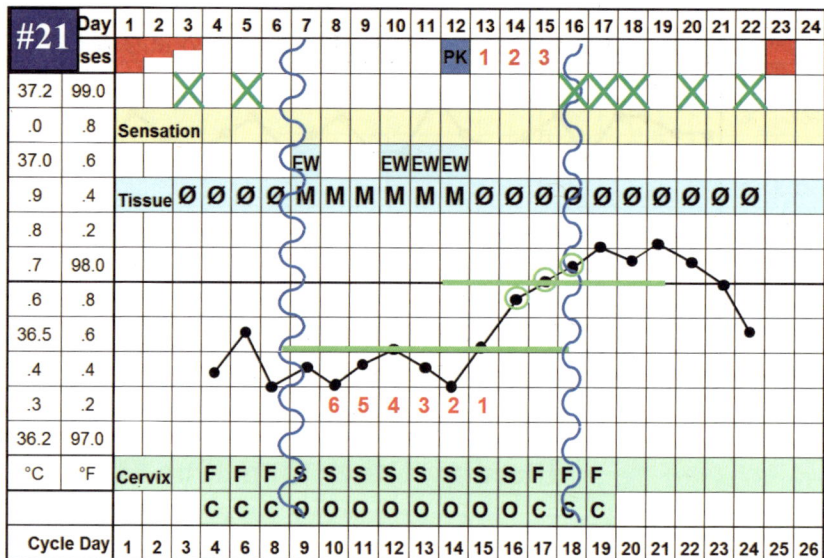

The 6-Day Rule has been 99.8+ percent effective in Dr. Roetzer's research. Identifying infertile days beyond Day 6 can also be highly effective.

Key Points:
- Identify the Completely Infertile Time using the Sympto-Thermal Rule.
- Beginners should follow the 6-5-0 Day Rule while studying their pattern of six last low temperatures and onset of mucus and cervical changes for 4 to 6 cycles.
- The phrase "6-Day Rule" always means "6-5-0 Day Rule."
- When assuming infertility beyond Days 5 or 6, follow the guidelines in the next section.

Assuming Infertility beyond Day 6

The 6-5-0 Day Rule is easy to apply. There are often more infertile days beyond Day 6, and many couples would like to take advantage of those days. Determining these infertile days takes the most experience, however. For effective NFP use, wait for 4 to 6 cycles before going beyond Day 6. At this point you might be able to apply the Early Dry Days Rule. There are other guidelines as well.

> **Wait for 4-6 cycles before going beyond Day 6 — become familiar with your cycle first.**

Early Dry Days Rule

With rare exception infertility lasts at least the first six days of the cycle, but after that, check carefully for the first sign of fertility. Chart to see if the day was Tissue-dry (Ø) and Sensation-dry (d) and the cervix was firm, low, closed, and dry. If so, you assume infertility at the *END OF THE DAY* once you are sure you were DRY all day first, by all the signs you checked. This is known as the "Early Dry Days Rule" (EDDR).

It is generally best to check at least two signs and to assume fertility **as soon as you notice any change**:

Observation	*Change*	
Tissue	from Ø to	M or EW-M
Sensation	from d to	$\frac{m}{M}$ or L
Cervix	from F,L,C,Ø to	S, H, O or M or EW-M

The first change may be by tissue, sensation, or cervix. It is helpful to avoid feminine hygiene products or clothing that may interfere with an accurate perception of sensation or that promote a continuous discharge (see pages 23 and 55). There are two helpful approaches to dealing with potential confusion from post-intercourse discharge (see page 47).

Effectiveness for the EDDR ranges between 97-99%. Effective use of this guideline requires excellent observing and charting as well as assuming fertility with the first sign by tissue, sensation, or cervix.

Crosscheck Dry Days against a Pattern of Six Last Low Temperatures

You might ask, "Can I confidently assume all the dry days beyond Day 6 to be infertile?" Maybe. Before assuming all these dry days infertile, look at your last 4 to 6 cycles and notice where the 6 low temperatures are marked (see Days 12-17 on chart #22) that helped you establish your Pre-Rise Baseline. Look at the tissue, sensation, and cervix signs. Do you notice a change away from dry to a more fertile sign on or before the 6th last low temperature in every cycle? In the cycle below, the first change was noticed on Day 10 by sensation, tissue, and cervix. If you do notice such a change every cycle, you can confidently assume all the dry days beyond Day 6 infertile at the end of the day by the Early Dry Days Rule.

A Change Before the 6th Last Low Temperature

Why the emphasis on a change on or before the final six lows? Research has established an identifiable "window of fertility." One study found that "the fertile period lasts about six days and ends on the day of ovulation."[4] Other studies correlate this window of fertility with the signs observed in NFP: the occurrence of pregnancies displays a bell curve pattern with a gradual increase occurring from the 6th last low temperature with a rapid rise and then a rapid drop-off by the first high temperature.[5] You can predict the onset of this window of fertility if you observe a change by tissue, sensation, or cervix occurring regularly just on or before the 6th last low temperature. This change providers an early sign of impending fertility.

---

4. Dunson, D., et al, "Changes with age in the level and duration of fertility in the menstrual cycle," *Human Reproduction*, 2002.
5. Gray, R.H., Kambic, R. T., "Epidemiological studies of natural family planning," *Human Reproduction*, 1988.

Distinguishing Arousal Fluid and Post-Intercourse Discharge

When applying the Early Dry Days Rule it is important to distinguish arousal fluid and post-intercourse discharge from cervical mucus. Arousal fluid is experienced by the woman as preparation for sexual intercourse. It is less lubricative and more watery than EW-M and it is specific to the time of arousal and disappears fairly quickly. It is best to determine one's fertility before arousal. Seminal fluid is similar to EW-M, so a woman needs to be able to evaluate the discharge after intercourse.

There are two guidelines which many women find helpful when trying to understand post-intercourse discharge. Each woman, however, needs to determine which will best suit her based on the observations she is making:

1. **One approach is "Alternate Dry Evenings."** The couple automatically assume the day after intercourse fertile, and if the day after that is again dry, it is infertile in the evening (take care to check and chart every day). Chart #23 displays the application of this rule.

Doing Kegel exercises helps to reduce any confusion. The Kegel exercise is also said to improve the woman's sexual pleasure as well as reduce the chances of developing weak pelvic muscles in later life. The simple procedure is as follows: urinate within an hour after intercourse (this aids against bladder infection). Then alternate between bearing down and doing 10-30 Kegel exercises to force seminal fluid down. A Kegel exercise involves repeatedly contracting and relaxing the pelvic floor muscles as if one were trying to stop and start urination. Wipe the vaginal entrance with toilet tissue until all the seminal fluid is removed. Each woman must learn how many Kegel exercises it takes for her to eliminate the seminal fluid. NOTE: This has no "contraceptive" value whatsoever; when fertility is present, sperm enter the cervix within seconds after intercourse.

2. **A second approach uses the "Cervix as Guide."** With this guideline, infertility is assumed by checking for a *firm, closed, and dry* cervix prior to intercourse: all days prior to a change can be considered infertile, any time of day. When a daily cervix check is being made, infertility can still be assumed any time of day until the start of the fertile time. This approach bypasses confusion at the vaginal entrance from fluids after intercourse. At least three cycles of experience with daily cervix checks is needed to learn the woman's pattern.

The Cervix as Guide

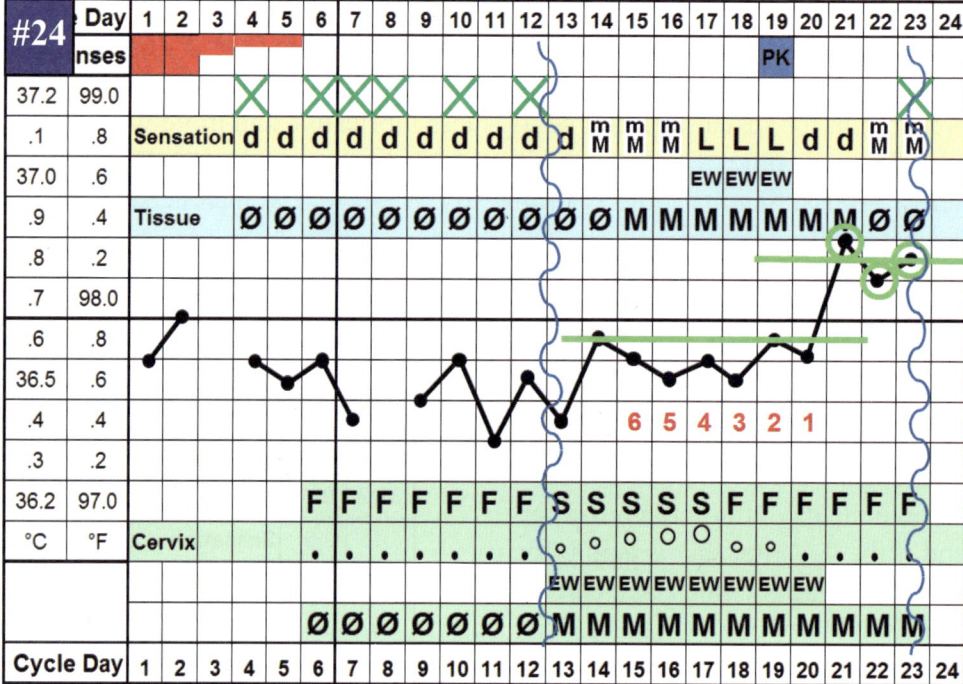

As shown in chart #24, once there is a change toward fertility by tissue, sensation, or cervix, the couple should assume fertility until the STR is fulfilled.

Steps for Applying the Early Dry Days Rule

- Assume yourself fertile after Days 5/6 for 4 to 6 cycles.
- Notice if you have a changing pattern by tissue, sensation, or cervix on or before the 6th last low temperature in every cycle. If not, you will need to follow other borderline rules.
- If you are dry and haven't started noticing any signs of fertility, assume yourself infertile in the evening.
- Follow either the Alternate Dry Evenings guideline or the Cervix as a Guide instructions for managing post-intercourse discharge.
- Once you observe fertile signs, assume yourself fertile until the Sympto-Thermal Rule (or some other rule your NFP Provider recommends).

— **ADVANCED RULES – Consult with your NFP Provider** —
Menses Fertile, Dry Days Afterwards Are Infertile

Some women occasionally have short cycles, but generally their cycles are longer than 23 days, for instance, women in premenopause. In the discussion of the 6-5-0 Day Rule, women who believed they had cycles less than 23 days are advised to follow a 0-Day Rule temporarily to evaluate the cycle pattern.

After a woman has established this pattern over the course of 4 to 6 cycles, she may be able to follow the Menses Fertile, Dry Days Infertile Rule. In such cases it is recommended that she observe during the light menstrual flow days for the presence of cervical mucus. Once she can observe she is dry by the tissue, sensation, or cervical signs, infertility can be assumed by applying the Alternate, Dry Evenings protocol. Once a fertility sign is present, assume fertility until a Sympto-Thermal Rule or other type of rule can be established.

6-5 Day Rule Borderline

Suppose you have only a short episode (2 to 4 days) of cervical mucus. What if you notice a change in signs only after the 6th last low temperature? If you are not charting all signs, for example, you haven't charted the cervix, you could begin charting the additional sign(s) and see if a consistent change is observed. If not, and it is important to avoid pregnancy, you could apply the 6-5 Day Rule and assume fertility immediately after Day 5 or 6, even if still dry, as shown here:

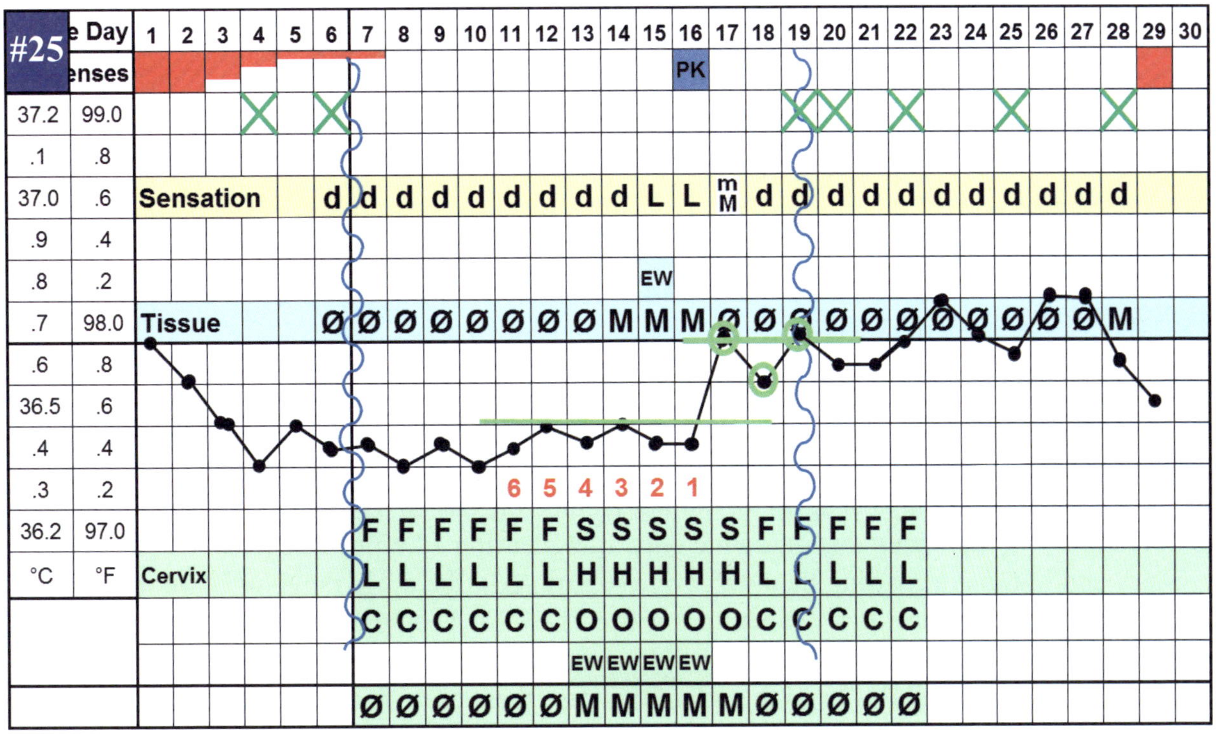

Earliest 6th Last Low Rule

Some couples who are avoiding pregnancy find it is psychologically easier to abstain after some fixed day instead of having intercourse until a "change" occurs by tissue, sensation, or cervix—particularly if the cervical mucus pattern is very short, there is a continuous discharge, or an ambiguous mucus pattern.

Going by Earliest 6th Last Low Rule with Short Mucus Episode

Another option for women with a limited mucus pattern is to follow the Earliest 6th Last Low Rule borderline. This requires a minimum of 12 charts, however.

Some couples use Day 6 as a borderline to mark the last day for intercourse. Another borderline rule for the "experienced NFP user" is "Earliest 6th Last Low = first fertile day." In other words, based on previous temperature history, you can calculate your last infertile day in the RIT. Dr. Gerd Döring's research findings showed a method-pregnancy rate of less than 1 percent using this rule even without a mucus crosscheck (99.7%). One would expect this rule to be equally or more effective when crosschecking with the cervical mucus, sensation, or cervix. You may apply this guideline in the following manner:

To follow this borderline rule, you need to have at least 12 charted biphasic cycles with the final 6 low temperatures marked on each one.

Find the earliest Cycle Day that is a 6th last low temperature in the diagram below:

Cycle Number	1	2	3	4	5	6	7	8	9	10	11	12
Cycle Day of 6th last low temperature	14	17	15	14	17	13	18	20	21	14	16	15

In the above diagram, the earliest 6th last low temperature occurs on Day 13 as seen on Cycle #6, which means the last infertile day by this guideline is Day 12. If there is an earlier occurrence of fertility signs or an earlier 6th last low temperature, the borderline would again be modified. Intercourse may occur up to, but not include the day of, the earliest 6th last low temperature. One can apply this guideline only after charting 12 biphasic cycles.

Mark and Maria are charting their 18th cycle (Chart #26); the cycle range is 32-36 days. So far, Maria's earliest 6th last low temperature was on Day 13. They drew a wavy vertical line before Day 13 indicating Day 12 was her last infertile day. They have decided to follow the Earliest 6th Last Low Rule — even though in this case there are a few more dry days.

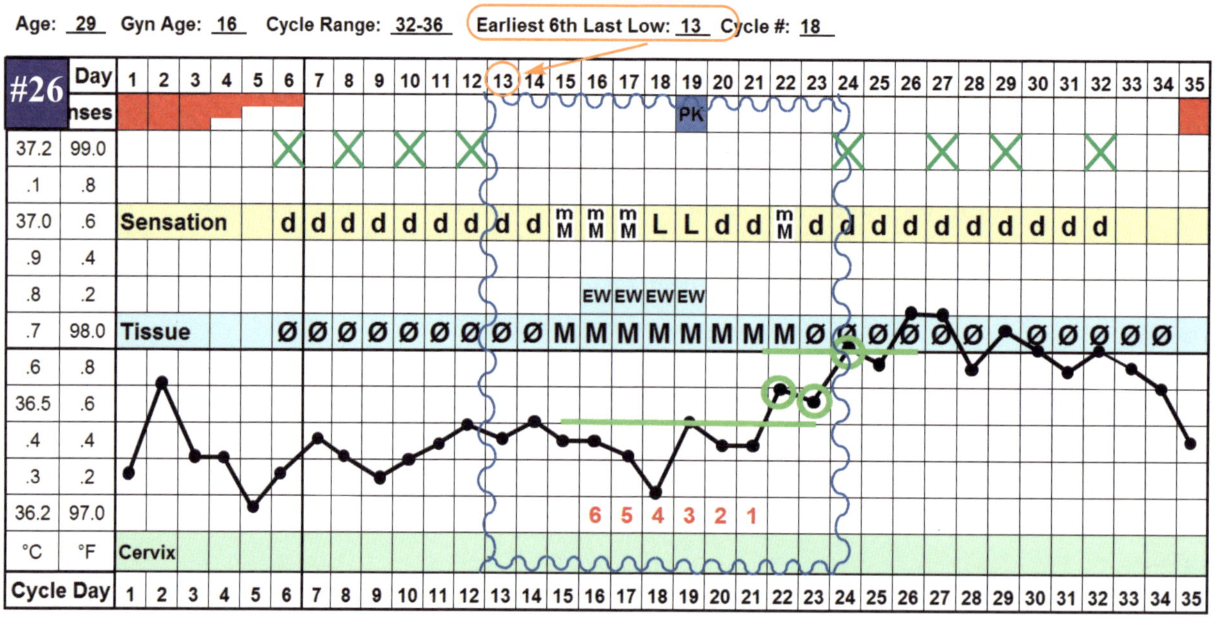

Maria's Cycle 25 (seven cycles later) has an earlier 6th last low temperature than ever before: Day 11. From the 26th cycle on, according the Earliest 6th Last Low Rule, Day 10 will be the last pre-ovulatory day for intercourse each cycle — unless an even earlier 6th last low temperature occurs.

In Cycle 26 cervical mucus began on Day 9. Mark and Maria assumed fertility at once, even though it was one day before the borderline day 10. When the cycle was complete, they knew the 6th last low temperature was not earlier than before, so they will keep Day 11 as the same borderline for next cycle. This borderline establishes the first fertile day.

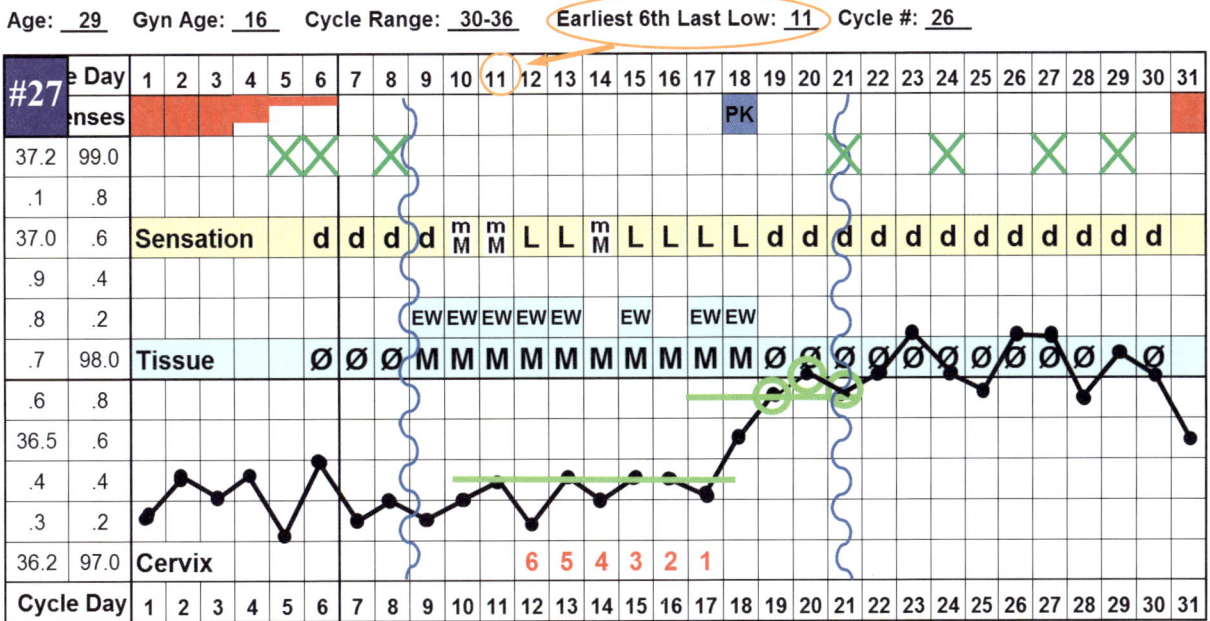

Sometimes a short cycle is due to a short high-temperature phase rather than an early ovulation. This is sometimes referred to as a short "luteal" phase as it reflects the time of the cycle when the corpus luteum is secreting progesterone after ovulation. If you have a very short cycle, look at the temperature pattern and notice where the final 6 low temperatures occur. If the 6 lows occur after Day 6 such as in the chart below, you may continue to apply the 6-Day Rule regardless of the cycle length.

Evaluating a Short Cycle with the Earliest 6th Last Low

The Earliest 6th Last Low Rule may sound like "calendar rhythm," but as given here, it is not. It is based on actual biphasic cycles. You know your true cycle lengths and whether or not bleeding is really menstrual. With the required 12 cycles, the information is predictive of future cycles. This guideline refines any "rhythm approach" in two ways:

1. By using the crosscheck for cervical mucus in case of early fertility.
2. By using the individual woman's temperature pattern instead of a fixed calculation.

The Earliest 6th Last Low Rule is a prudent extension of the infertile time beyond Day 6 and is highly effective. In typical cycles, borderline rules are more reassuring and more effective than using all the dry days before the start of cervical mucus.

Shortcut Approach

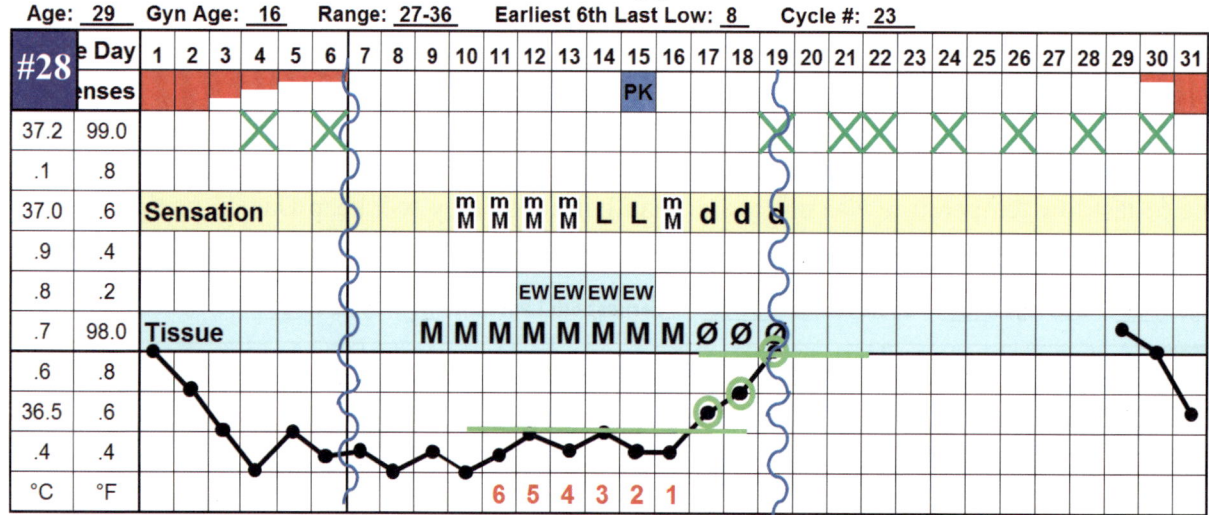

Some couples using NFP wish to reduce charting to a minimum but maintain high effectiveness. This is possible for the experienced NFP user. For example, a couple can start charting temperature from about Day 6, or when the cervical mucus starts and continues, until the 4th encircled reading. If the woman is going to make infrequent cervical mucus observations, the couple should abstain after Day 6 or the Earliest 6th Last Low Borderline.

In Chart 28, the couple abstains after Day 6 until the Sympto-Thermal Rule is fulfilled. The woman carefully observes the cervical mucus to determine Peak Day. She likes to take a few temperatures about the expected time of menstruation, to verify the highs and the drop in temperature that warns her of the onset of the menstrual period.

Some women, however, find that a "routine, automatic, daily habit" of cervical mucus, sensation, cervix, and temperature observations is for them easier to live with than remembering again each cycle to chart carefully. You need to decide for yourself what fits your needs and lifestyle.

- Find the best way to communicate the onset of the fertile time with your spouse.
- Identify 2 or 3 positive ways to manage abstinence so that it helps enhance your relationship.

Key Points:

- After charting 4 to 6 cycles, infertility after Day 5 or 6 may be determined by the Early Dry Days Rule. This involves crosschecking tissue, sensation, and cervix in relationship to the earliest 6th last low temperature. Infertility is assumed evenings only.
- If a change in tissue, sensation, or cervix does not always occur on or before the 6th last low temperature, don't assume all the early dry days are infertile. Follow a borderline rule instead.
- It is best to restrict intercourse to the evenings of dry days during the pre-ovulatory Relatively Infertile Time.
- Develop skills for identifying and managing post-intercourse discharge.
- The Earliest 6th Last Low Rule can be applied as a borderline rule after 12 biphasic cycles.
- A shortcut approach to charting usually means more days of abstinence.

The Basic Mucus Rule
(For use with long cycles or during times of transition)

Some people believe that NFP can't be used with irregular cycles or during breastfeeding, premenopause, or while recovering from hormonal contraceptive use. They are confusing NFP with Calendar Rhythm. Modern NFP allows the woman to use the information from the tissue-paper, sensation, and cervix to apply the Basic Mucus Rule (BMR), or one of its variations, in accord with advice from her NFP Provider. During typical cycling, however, use of the BMR may not yield the same effectiveness as waiting for the Sympto-Thermal Rule to confirm the Completely Infertile Time.

The Basic Mucus Rule (BMR) is: once there's a change from dry, assume fertility until Peak and for 4 days afterward. If the 4th day after Peak Day is dry, you can assume infertility in the evening on Peak + 4.

If avoiding pregnancy while using the BMR, it is important to *continue checking carefully* for cervical mucus and cervix changes. Don't become lax. Continue to check and chart until you are sure you are in the Completely Infertile Time by the STR. The chart below applies the BMR to a case of a long, erratic cycle pattern prior to the application of the Sympto-Thermal Rule. This woman has a cycle range of 38-65 days (See Chart #29). Upon the advice of her NFP Provider she is applying the BMR to episodes of cervical mucus which occur before the Sympto-Thermal Rule can be applied.

> **Peak Day**
> Peak Day is the last day of any trait of the most fertile sign, usually EW-M or L (the last day that any T, OT, G, 1" or L was present). If no EW-M or L could be observed, Peak Day is the last day of any mucus (M) or moistness (^m_M).

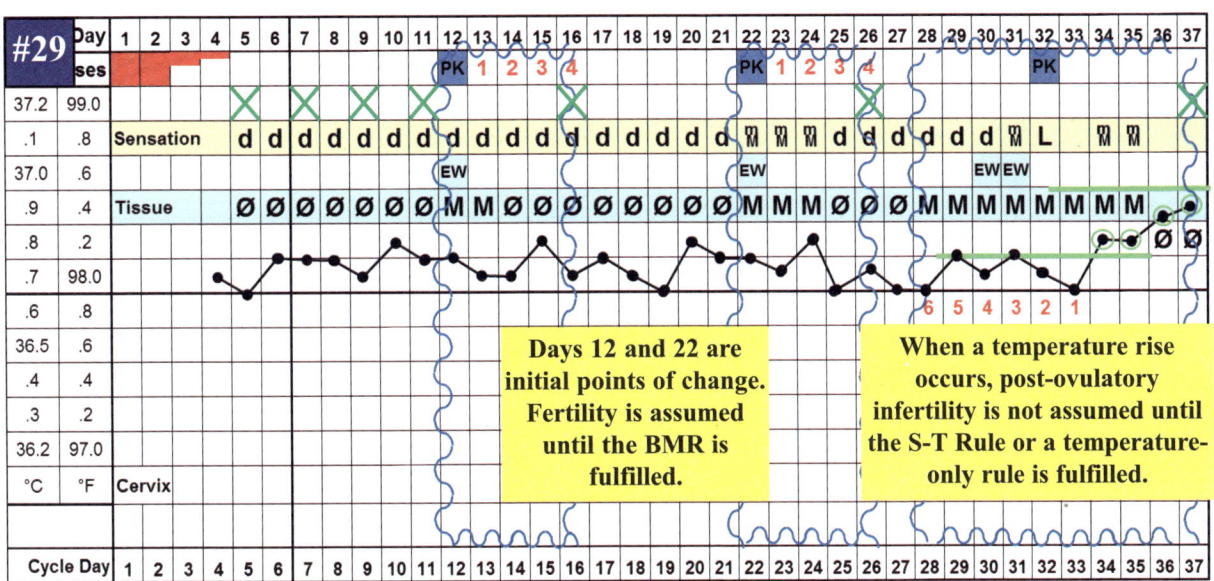

Careful Charting
Days 12 and 22 are initial points of change.

The BMR is a guideline for the Relatively Infertile Time. You need to observe your fertility signs consistently throughout the day. Infertility is assumed evenings only of dry days. Dry days during the Pk+3 count are considered fertile.

As long as the temperatures remain low, don't assume Completely Infertile Time after a Peak+4 count. You may be experiencing multiple Peak Days which aren't associated with ovulation. You need to continue to observe for another episode of cervical mucus. Until you observe a sustained temperature rise, you probably have not ovulated. The Pk+4 count in the chart below is not accompanied with a sustained temperature rise. In such a case, the M on Day 20 and the bleeding on Days 21 and 22 must be considered fertile.

Non-menstrual Bleeding Is Always Considered Fertile

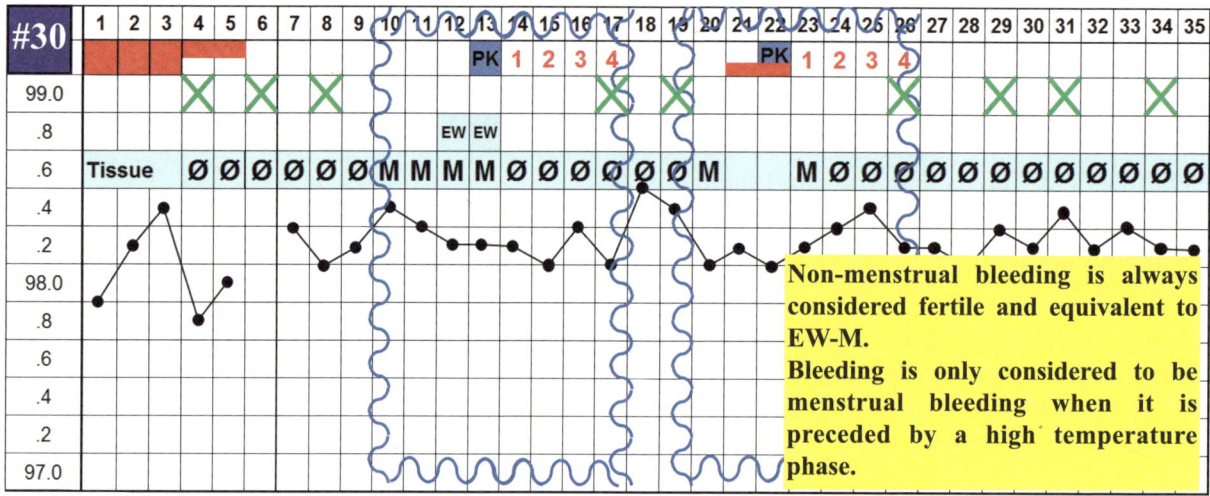

Non-menstrual bleeding is always considered fertile and equivalent to EW-M.
Bleeding is only considered to be menstrual bleeding when it is preceded by a high temperature phase.

The 6-5 Day Rule Doesn't Apply without a Temperature Rise. The reason for this is that ovulation bleeding with intermenstrual pain may seem similar to menstruation. Your true menstrual period will have a temperature rise one to two weeks beforehand.

Always consider non-menstrual bleeding fertile, as if cervical mucus, in case it is ovulation bleeding. Only if you take your temperature will you know for sure if a sustained temperature rise occurred before the bleeding or not. Without the temperature pattern on the second half of the chart 31, the bleeding on Day 33-35 must be considered fertile.

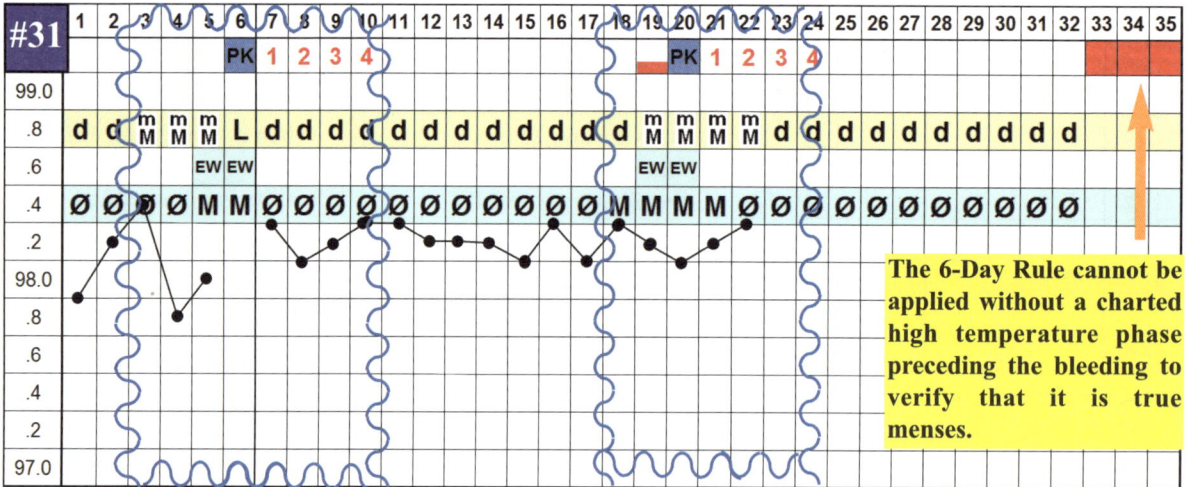

The 6-Day Rule cannot be applied without a charted high temperature phase preceding the bleeding to verify that it is true menses.

When bleeding is observed, apply the 6-5 Day Rule only if there was a sustained temperature rise beforehand. Otherwise, assume ovulation is yet to come, and consider all bleeding fertile, as if EW-M, and apply a Peak+4 count:

Don't fall into Rhythm thinking! When you aren't taking your temperature, even the usual bleeding at the usual time after a mucus pattern should be considered fertile and the Basic Mucus Rule (Pk+4) applied.

When cycling hasn't begun after childbirth, or when cycles become very long, some women become anxious because there's "never any mucus" or because they have mucus but it "never changes." That is precisely the pattern needed to identify infertility: the unchanging symptom (whether dry or a continuous discharge) means the ovaries are at rest, the body is not yet preparing an egg for ovulation.

Continuous Discharge. A woman can apply the Basic Mucus Rule even if she has a continuous discharge. To do so she has to find out what is "as if dry" for her. This takes conscientious charting and the help of her NFP Provider.

Chart the traits of any mucus discharge (color, amount, stretch, tissue glide, sensation, how often observed during the day).

Rule out any pathology by eliminating irritant factors that may cause continuous or confusing discharge and by consulting with your health care provider.

By counting an unchanging discharge as if dry, and any change from it as fertile, the Basic Mucus Rule can be applied even when the woman has no dry days. This may have a higher pregnancy rate than if the basic pattern were dry. Crosschecking for a firm, low, closed cervix can be a confirmation of infertility during an "unchanging" pattern of continuous discharge.

A consistently low temperature provides reassurance that pregnancy has not occurred. Of course, when a temperature rise finally occurs, the Completely Infertile Time can be identified.

Missed Period. When a woman says, "I missed my period this month," she is really having a long cycle – a delayed ovulation. This occurs more frequently during stress, after childbirth, and during adolescence or premenopause. It is important to stick with the NFP guidelines one has learned. This means to wait until the STR is met before assuming one is in the Completely Infertile Time or, if not cycling, to use the Basic Mucus Rule as advised by one's NFP Provider. For the highest effectiveness, couples in typical cycles should not apply the BMR in an isolated stress cycle. Rather the couple should wait for the STR to be fulfilled. If pregnancy is the reason for a "late period," then there will also be a high-temperature phase of more than 18 days. As long as the temperature readings remain at the low level, ovulation is delayed. Remember: Menstruation won't occur until about two weeks after ovulation, at the end of the high-temperature phase.

Key Points:
- The Basic Mucus Rule is a guideline for the Relatively Infertile Time. The most common application is after childbirth or during premenopause. You need to observe during the day. Infertility is assumed evenings only on dry days. Dry days during Pk+3 are considered fertile.
- When a woman has typical cycles, the STR would be preferred over the BMR.
- If you haven't observed a sustained temperature rise, you probably have not ovulated.
- When bleeding is observed, apply the 6-5 Day Rule only if there was a sustained temperature rise first.
- Application of the Basic Mucus Rule to a non-changing continuous discharge is best done with the advice of an NFP Provider.

Temperature-Only Rules

There are times when a couple may need to rely on a temperature-only guideline. For example, if a woman experiences a yeast infection, has a confusing cervical mucus pattern, or has no mucus days, temperature-only rules are very helpful. The high-temperature phase indicates that ovulation has occurred.

There is a note of caution to women who want to consistently apply a temperature-only rule. Without knowing one's cervical mucus pattern, a woman who experiences a long cycle because of stress, premenopause, or childbirth, would not be familiar with or confident of her mucus observations if she has relied solely on the temperature. The strength of the Sympto-Thermal Method is in the variety of signs and the ability to crosscheck the information. This means at times giving precedence to one sign over another.

When the cervical mucus sign is disturbed or absent, the following two temperature-only guidelines may be helpful: the "Mean Temperature Rule" and the "Basal Body Temperature Rule" (BBT Rule). If there is a shallow overall rise or if the temperatures in the current cycle are missing or disturbed, the "Mean Temperature Rule" would be more applicable. The BBT Rule is most helpful when there is a dramatic temperature rise.

Using a "Temperature-Only" rule requires proper temperature taking. Be sure to note all disturbances. A crosscheck for a firm, closed cervix may confirm the temperature rise if external cervical mucus checking is impossible or inconclusive.

Both of these temperature-only rules are highly effective for identifying post-ovulatory infertility: 99.9%. It is still possible to apply the 6-5 Day Rule with the subsequent knowledge when applying temperature-only rules as well.

The general principle behind virtually all temperature rules in use throughout the world is "3 highs establish infertility." Various additional requirements like "wait until evening," "wait until 3 highs after Peak Day," "wait until the temperatures are a certain amount higher," or "wait an additional day" have been developed to reduce occasional unintended pregnancies occurring when a less strict rule is used. The most versatile and effective single rule is the Sympto-Thermal Rule (see page 35).

The Mean (or Average) Temperature Rule. Use the mean or average temperature of one cycle as the dividing line between low and high temperatures for the following cycle. This rule is helpful if the current cycle has disturbed temperatures, but the one before it was normal. For instance, in Chart #33, (see page 58) the woman was ill and had several disturbed temperatures due to a fever during the critical days of fertility; that is, a Pre-Rise Baseline could not be set. In this case, however, chart data from her previous cycle can be used to establish a mean or average dividing line for Chart #33.

Here's how it works. **First Cycle (Chart 32):** Add up all undisturbed temperature readings and divide by the number of readings. The undisturbed chart must have at least 75 percent of the temperatures charted, with missing or disturbed temperatures evenly distributed throughout the cycle. There are 29 undisturbed temperatures below. When the temperatures were added together it came to 2932.3 (degrees)/30 (days). This yielded a mean or average temperature of 97.74°F. Compute to the nearest hundredth of a degree, and use this as a "dividing line" for the following cycle, as shown on the next page. A calculator helps.

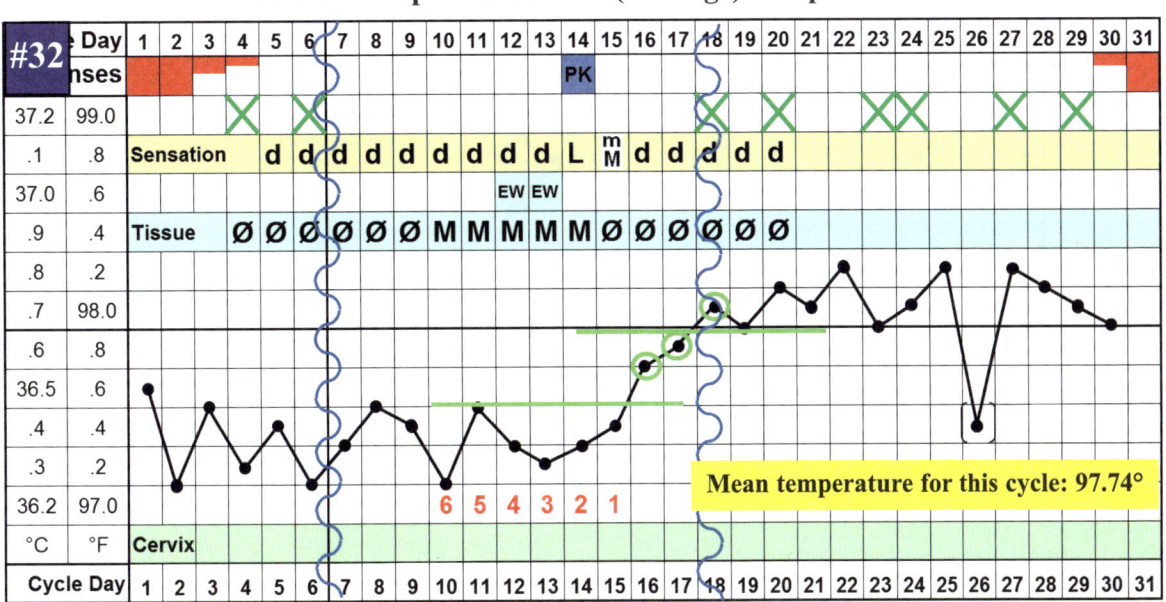

How to Compute the Mean (Average) Temperature

Second Cycle (Chart 33): The temperatures on Days 10 and 11 of Chart #33 are disturbed due to an illness. In order to establish a Pre-Rise Baseline, there needs to be at least 5 undisturbed temperatures. With only 4 temperatures, it would be impossible to apply the Sympto-Thermal Rule. The mean temperature (97.74°F) from the previous, undisturbed cycle, becomes the dividing line for the next cycle. Starting with morning on the 4th day in a row on or above the "dividing line," assume the Completely Infertile Time until the end of the cycle. The temperature taking conditions (time and way) must remain constant from one cycle to the next. The Completely Infertile Time begins in the morning of the 4th temperature in a row on or above the mean (average) temperature. If a temperature drops below the mean, the count must be restarted.

This approach is helpful when evaluating an unusual cycle or if you cannot determine Peak Day. The Mean Temperature Rule may require more days of abstinence than with the STR.

Applying the Mean Temperature Rule (From Previous Cycle)

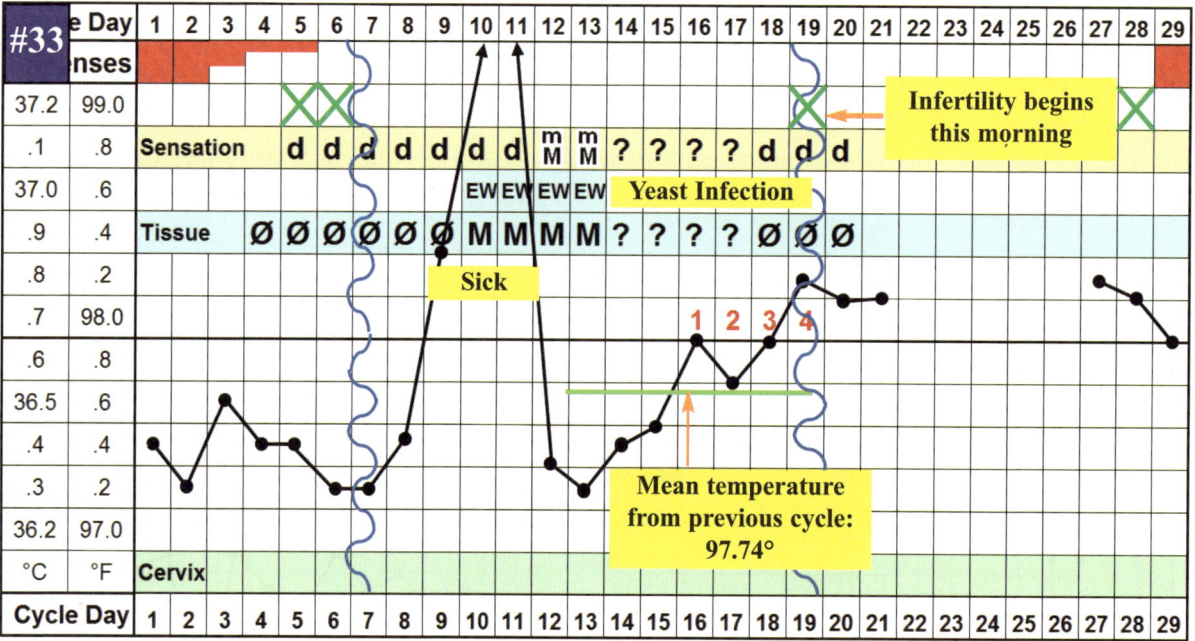

THE BBT RULE. Look for 3 high temperatures in a row all 0.4°F or more (= 0.2°C or more) above the Pre-Rise Baseline. Mark these temperatures "1, 2, 3." The Completely Infertile Time begins in the evening on the 3rd consecutive high temperature. All three high temperatures must be 0.4°F or more above the PRB, and they must be consecutive. The temperatures on Days 18 and 19 don't count because Day 19 dropped below the FTSL.

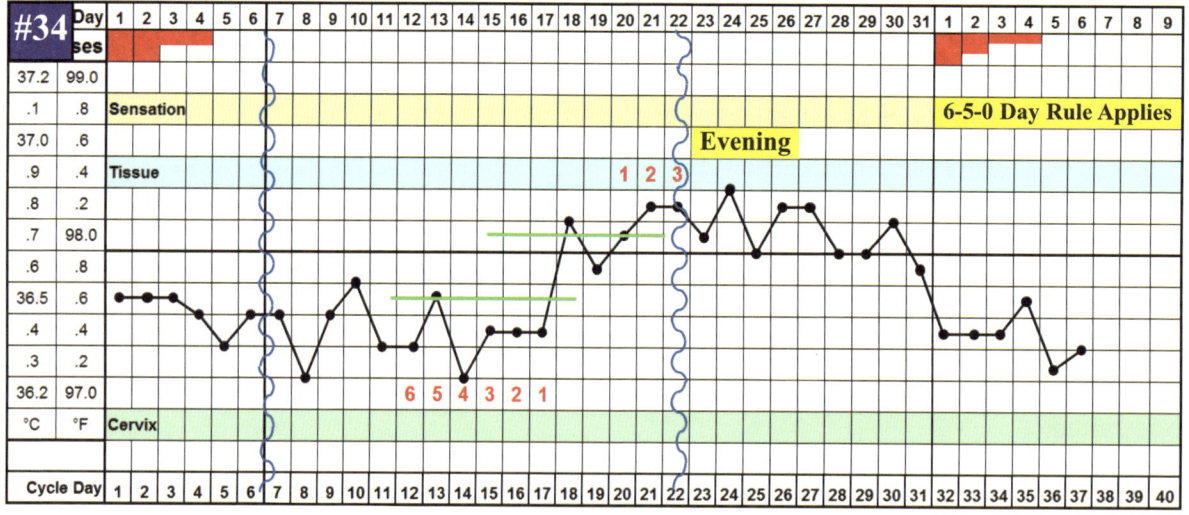

BBT Rule

The challenge with the BBT Rule is that it can only be applied to about a third of cycles. Try not to confuse this rule with the less strict temperature rise requirement of the Sympto-Thermal Rule (STR). With the crosscheck found in the STR, a more liberal temperature rise requirement still yields a high effectiveness. When only using one sign, such as just the temperature, one must be stricter with the application.

Key Points:
- The Mean Rule and BBT Temperature can help to positively identify the CIT when tissue, sensation, and cervix data don't allow interpretation with STR.
- With long or erratic cycles, and during breastfeeding or premenopause, the extended RIT needs to be interpreted with the use of the EDDR and the BMR or one of its variants.

Stress

It is well known that stress can affect the human body. At different times in their lives, people can successfully manage varying degrees of stress. In addition, a certain amount of stress is beneficial to people.

People generally think of stress as negative. Stress, however, may be pleasant or unpleasant; physical or emotional. Some causes of stress might be: death in the family, wedding, a new baby, new job, moving, visitors, major decisions, illness, accidents, holidays, school, travel, dieting, excessive demands at work, or strenuous exercise.

When understanding the impact of stress and the menstrual cycle, one needs to know that it may affect a woman's menstrual cycle but does not necessarily do so. If stress does affect the cycle, it will do so in one of two ways. Ovulation may be delayed and the woman may notice more than one mucus Peak. Or a shortened high-temperature phase may occur (a shortened luteal phase).

Eliminating unnecessary stress will certainly help. Chronic underrest, poor or erratic eating habits, and inadequate exercise may lead to poor health and be reflected in the menstrual cycle pattern. Stress factors also have a cumulative effect. For example, changing one's job may result in a small amount of stress, but when compounded with relocating to a different city, the net effect is considerably greater.

People under stress are often unable to accurately assess their own situation. When a group of situations arises in one's life, each added upon another, the person is often doing all he or she can just to survive. Stepping out of oneself, recognizing the situation, and saying, "Hmm, it appears I have taken on too much. What can I change?" is often beyond one's ability when under stress.

Sometimes a woman doesn't realize she is in a stress situation, but her husband may recognize it. She needs to listen to his observations. Dr. Roetzer's first advice to husbands concerned about extended abstinence in confusing cycles is "Be kind to your wife!" Positive steps to managing stress include a proper regimen of sleep and relaxation, a proper diet with additional vitamins, regular exercise, and prayer.

With that in mind, if anything seems stressful to you, note it on your chart. It may or may not affect the cycle. If it does, note how.

CHAPTER FOUR: ACHIEVING PREGNANCY

NFP is true family planning. A couple desiring to achieve a pregnancy can use the same information they used to avoid pregnancy to identify the most fertile time: the days of best quality mucus and the days of maximum "SHOW" cervix (soft, high, open, wet [M], or EW-M) until the first high temperature.

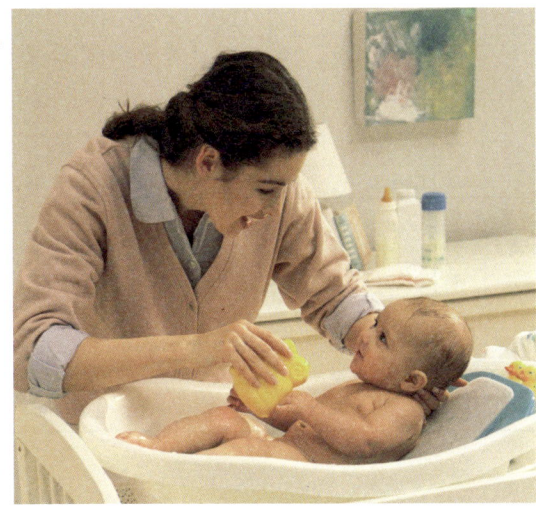

Some people believe they need to just stop avoiding pregnancy and they'll automatically achieve one. This may or may not be the case. Even a couple with "normal" fertility may take from six to twelve cycles of having focused intercourse to become pregnant. Focused intercourse means consistently having sexual intercourse on the best fertile days. And though it may seem frustrating, there is no need to worry if pregnancy does not occur in the first few cycles. Keep observing and charting. If after six to twelve cycles you are still not pregnant, check with your health care provider. Be sure to bring in your charts; however, you may want to review your charts ahead of time with your NFP Provider.

NFP can help identify the fertile time when it occurs. Though NFP can't cure infertility, at least it won't cause infertility, as sometimes happens with hormonal contraceptives or the IUD.

Identifying Pregnancy. The cervical mucus pattern and cervix may vary in early pregnancy. Temperature taking, however, can be one of the earliest and most accurate pregnancy indicators: once you have 18-20 high temperature readings, it is 99 percent certain you are pregnant. In addition, a common observation is for the woman to notice a second rise in her temperatures to yet another level around the time she expects her menstrual period as on Day 29 on Chart 35.

The Importance of Prenatal Care. The relatively few complications and deaths for the mother and infant are due almost totally to the early and constant care pregnant women should receive. Even while you are thinking about becoming pregnant, but definitely as soon as you know you are pregnant (18-20 high temperatures), take special care to get proper rest, nutrition, and pre-natal vitamins (e.g., folic acid significantly reduces the incidence of spina bifida and other birth defects), and make an appointment with a health care provider. Avoid all medication not approved by your doctor for use during pregnancy. And avoid smoking, marijuana and other illegal drugs, caffeine products, and alcohol — it is best for mother and child.

Setting the Due Date. Find the calendar day around which Peak Day and the first high temperature occurs; then add 9 months, and subtract one week. Be sure to stand by your charting information on this matter when visiting your physician. Pregnancy does not necessarily occur two weeks after menstruation, so a due date calculation based on your last menstrual period could be significantly in error if your cycles vary from the 28 day norm. This is of particular importance if a woman has irregular cycles and then needs to schedule a Caesarean section.

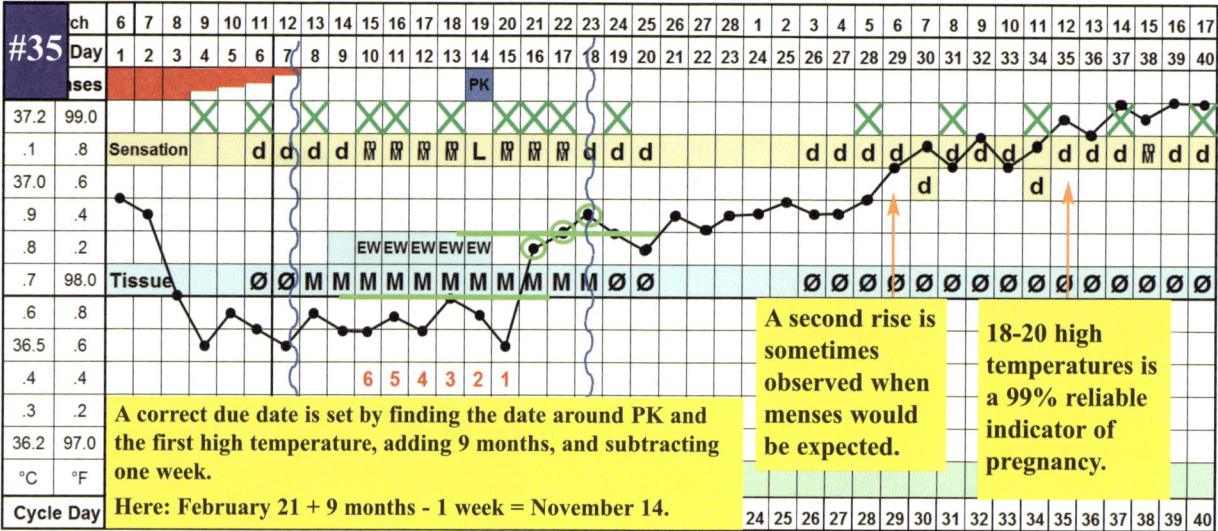

Why do some people have difficulty achieving a pregnancy? About 20 percent of couples suffer from some form of infertility. Thankfully, a significant number of couples do go on to achieve a pregnancy through routine treatment. Infertility can be related to the man or the woman or a combination of both. For example, the man may have a low sperm count or the woman may ovulate infrequently or have a blockage in her fallopian tubes. Be sure to review any medications or herbal treatments you or your spouse may be taking as well as any home or workplace environmental issues that may impact fertility. There are numerous reasons for infertility. Some infertility is related to disease and some reflects the biological clock ticking. Men and women are marrying later and delaying childbirth. Male fertility is generally constant from the onset of puberty until old age; however, recent evidence shows men, too, experience some decrease in fertility over time. The woman's fertility is age dependent and begins to decline around age 30 and then more rapidly decreases from age 35 until menopause.

NFP and Sex Selection. The sex of the child is determined by the chromosome from the sperm. For most couples, there is a 50 percent chance of conceiving a boy or a girl. One theory claims there will be a slightly greater chance of conceiving a boy if intercourse occurs around Peak Day and a slightly greater chance of conceiving a girl if intercourse happens only at the beginning of the fertile time followed by abstinence until the Completely Infertile Time. The little controlled evidence available from a few small studies is conflicting. A more thoughtful position might be to gratefully accept the joys of the child you are given, regardless of its gender.

What can you learn from the NFP chart? Some women experience a short "luteal" (high-temperature) phase. This is indicative of poor ovulation. A short luteal phase is one in which the high-temperature phase is less than eight days.

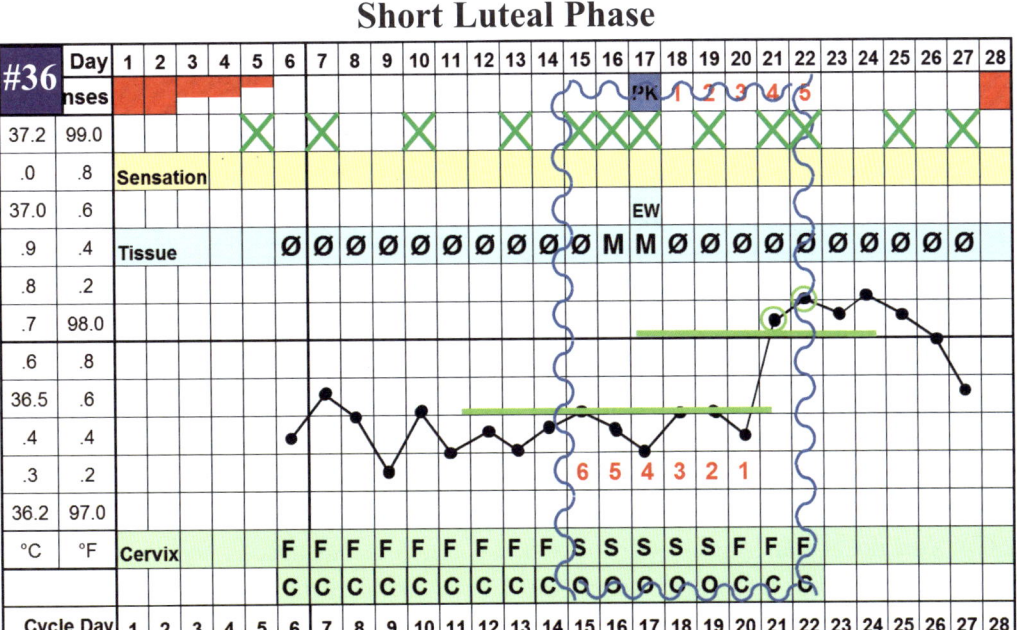

Some couples will find that the temperature and cervical mucus signs do not align on some of their charts. This can be reflective of a hormonal imbalance making it difficult to conceive.

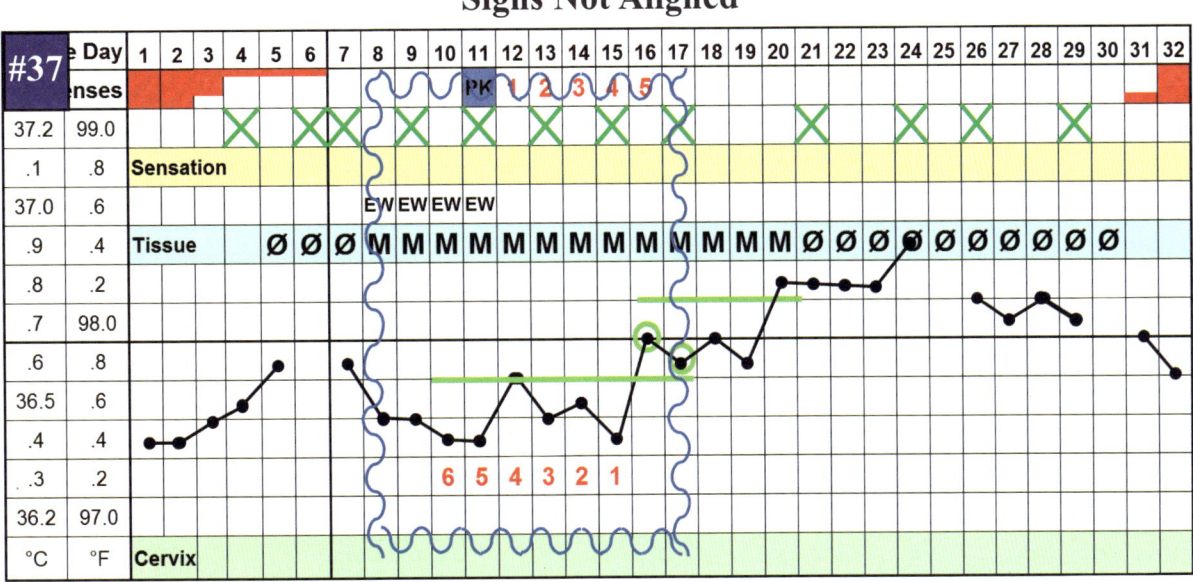

Sometimes women will experience cycles with little or no cervical mucus. This can be due to cervical surgery, hormonal imbalance, or other factors.

Scant Cervical Mucus Pattern

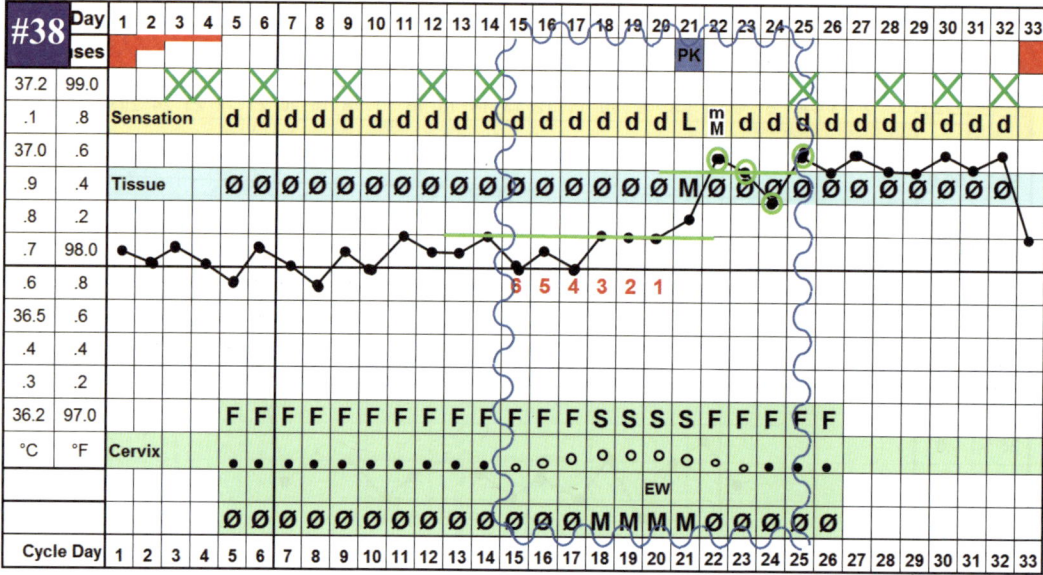

What can you do? Charting allows you to see if the cervical mucus and temperature signs that occur reflect a typical fertility pattern. Lifestyle issues can make a difference. For example, women who are underweight with very low levels of body fat will cease to ovulate — and probably not "menstruate." Overweight women will experience higher levels of infertility. Thyroid imbalances can affect fertility. A basal body temperature level consistently below 97.0°F (32.2°C) is an indication of low thyroid (hypothyroid). Stress is certainly a factor which affects one's well being and one's fertility. Smoking cigarettes and marijuana are known to impact the fertility of men and women as well as result in increased miscarriages and low birthweight babies. An ingredient called guaifansein found in some cough expectorants does promote the production of cervical mucus for those women who have little or none. Vitamins, especially B complex, minerals, and herbs such as Vitex have assisted some couples in achieving a pregnancy (consult with a professional on this matter). An excellent resource book in this area is *Fertility, Cycles, and Nutrition* by Marilyn Shannon. Progesterone augmentation can help women who have a short or otherwise inadequate high temperature phase. Another excellent book related to the benefits of natural progesterone to assist in achieving a pregnancy is entitled *What Your Doctor May Not Tell You about Menopause* by John R. Lee, M.D., (don't let the title put you off). You can also do an Internet search for"bioidentical hormones, or "natural progesterone," or speak with a healthcare provider to learn more.

Women who have discontinued hormonal contraceptives such as birth control pills, patches, injectables, and implants experience difficulty achieving pregnancy or an increased incidence of miscarriage for at least the first 6 to 12 months. The average return of menstrual periods for women discontinuing *DepoProvera* is 10 months - actual fertility may be delayed even longer. Physical conditions such as endometriosis make achieving a pregnancy more difficult. Breastfeeding women, even after cycling resumes, may have more difficulty conceiving until weaning is complete. Some women who are correctly diagnosed with polycystic ovarian syndrome have successfully achieved a pregnancy after receiving corrective treatment for their insulin levels.

Male Fertility Issues. Since the woman is the one who becomes pregnant or not, the emphasis tends to be on her. Obviously, the husband can suffer some form of infertility. It is estimated that one-third of infertility cases are female related, one-third are male related, and one-third are a combination of both. It's not a matter of blame, rather the approach should initially be on trying to find out the source(s) of infertility. Basic techniques to assess female fertility have been discussed using NFP observations. Assessing male fertility requires doing a semen analysis. The moral solution to obtaining a semen sample for analysis is through intercourse using a perforated condom. Special "male factor" condoms are used which do not affect the sperm cells. Another way to evaluate the husband's sperm quality, the woman's cervical mucus, and the interaction of the two is through a post-coital test. This procedure requires the woman make a doctor visit immediately after intercourse to assess the post-intercourse fluids. The best time to conduct this test is during the Possibly Fertile Time when the best quality mucus is present.

Achieving: Lifestyle and Fertility	
Taking care of one's health is a given after a pregnancy is confirmed. There are factors that contribute to the fertility health of both men and women.	
Alcohol consumption	Avoid/Limited Use
Smoking	Avoid
Marijuana/drugs	Avoid
Caffeine products	Avoid/Limited Use
Stress	Minimize
Diet high in refined carbohydrates	Avoid/Limited
Over or underweight	Avoid
Excessive driving or hot tub use for men	Avoid
For details and the sources check this website: http://www.usccb.org/prolife/issues/nfp/cmrsf03.shtml#6	

There are a number of possible sources of male infertility. A varicocele, which is a dilation or swelling of the veins that drain the testicle, is a common source and can be surgically treated. Hormonal factors are another. Environmental factors, diseases, medical treatments, and lifestyle issues (such as STDs, marijuana, tobacco, and alcohol use) can contribute to infertility. Nutritional products, such as ProXeed, have been found to improve male fertility if this is the problem (see www.proxeed.com). Lifestyle changes can help.

Assisting Pregnancy. The ovulation process is often assisted with Clomiphene Citrate (Clomid, Serophone) as well as other agents which stimulate FSH and LH production. But Thomas Hilgers, M.D., says of Clomiphene Citrate that "it is a medication that *inhibits cervical mucus production*." Since it is a strong drug, "low doses of Clomiphene actually stimulate ovarian function quite well," and do the least impairment to the cervical mucus factor for fertility.[6] The reason for taking Clomiphene Citrate or some other related product is to induce ovulation. NFP users can easily identify the occurrence of a biphasic temperature pattern as a good indicator of ovulation. If ovulation induction is advised by a physician, refer to your chart or request additional ovulation assessment before taking Clomiphene Citrate. It is a matter of problem-solving the condition accurately. A study comparing natural technology compared with "assisted reproductive technology" including in vitro fertilization found comparable births.[7]

---
6. Hilgers, Thomas, M.D., "The Medical Approach of Natural Family Planning," Pope Paul VI Institute Press, 1991.
7. Stanford, J. B., MD, MSPH, Parnell, T. A., MD, & Boyle, P. C., MB (2008). Outcomes From Treatment of Infertility With Natural Procreative Technology in an Irish General Practice. *Journal of American Board of Family Medicine*, 375-384.

Progesterone is used once the Peak Day plus high-temperature phase has been established to supplement deficient progesterone levels or to support pregnancy in women who have experienced a previous miscarriage. Be sure to do your research to understand the difference between natural progesterone and synthetic progestins. Women may require other forms of natural progesterone and should work with their healthcare provider. (More information on natural progesterone can be found at http://www.healingedge.net/store/page232.html.) Medical personnel who have received training through NaProTECHNOLOGY or FertilityCare are especially skilled in such treatment (http://www.naprotechnology.com/). These are healthcare providers who are especially supportive of NFP and understand the dynamics of the female fertility cycle.

NFP users know a great deal more about their own fertility than most women do, so it is important to use that information to your advantage. For example, a physician may want to check a woman's progesterone level through a blood test. She would know to ask to have it assessed during her high temperature phase.

There are many "high tech" alternatives to identifying and treating infertility. When one enters into the domain of the generation of life, there are certain moral issues involved. For a brief discussion of this matter please refer to page 110.

Dealing with the Emotional Challenges of Infertility.
Emotional issues may be especially difficult if a couple is experiencing "unexplained infertility"–infertility for which no apparent reason can be found. Some common emotional responses to infertility include disbelief and denial, anger, guilt and blame, sadness and depression, hopelessness, loss of control, and isolation. These struggles may be compounded by the fact that partners may be "out of sync" in their emotional responses at any given time.

Each person must take responsibility for his or her feelings. You are separate individuals and may respond differently–both in behavior and emotions. Try to identify your feelings and share them with your spouse. He or she may truly not know what you are thinking or feeling or what you need. Be willing to accept the other's feelings; understanding does not mean that you agree.

Protect and build the intimacy and commitment in your relationship. Intercourse may be difficult because it can be a reminder of what's not happening – it may seem pointless if pregnancy isn't possible. Be sure to express your affection for your partner – verbally and physically or through acts that will be meaningful to him or her. Remember that your marriage relationship is central to any family relationships you may have. You married each other out of love and a desire to share a life together. Children may have been a warmly anticipated part of that life, but only a part. Build your relationship. Strengthen it. Make time for fun together.

Remember what brought you together in the first place. When thinking of others outside your marriage relationship, help them help you. Again, they truly may not know what you are thinking or feeling or what you need from them. Have realistic expectations. No matter how close your friend, no matter how much your family loves you, there will be times that someone is not there for you.

Counseling may be helpful in dealing with guilt or blame. It can help you deal with any depression. It is a time to address differences in opinion about treatment options or whether to consider adoption. Counseling can help you find a renewed sense of self and develop coping skills. Support groups with guidelines congruent with your ethical beliefs may also be helpful by letting you get to know others in your situation.

Fertility is often taken for granted. There is often the expectation that as soon as pregnancy is desired, it will be achieved. Couples may not have ever given serious thought to infertility before facing it themselves. While it is a crisis experience of loss, couples working through infertility may be strengthened as individuals and as a couple.

> **"The way to plan the family is natural family planning, not contraception. In destroying the power of giving life, through contraception, a husband or wife is doing something to self, and so it destroys the gift of life in him or her."**
> **Blessed Mother Teresa**

CHAPTER FIVE: SPECIAL CIRCUMSTANCES

Discontinuing Hormonal Contraceptives

The choice of hormonal contraceptives includes the Pill, the Patch, implants, rings, and injectables, and in some cases the IUD (intrauterine device). Each form of hormonal contraception is somewhat different. The list of contraceptives changes with some being removed from the market and new ones added. The descriptions below represent those available at the time of printing.

Hormonal Contraceptives such as the Birth Control Pill and the Contraceptive Patch
The information in this section applies to the following hormonal contraceptives:

- The traditional birth control pill actually is comprised of dozens of types of pills with numerous chemical and dosage variations. The hallmark for this drug is that women usually experience a monthly bleeding.
- There is an extended pill, such as the product *Seasonale,* which is taken for three month intervals. When it is taken the woman is supposed to experience only four menstrual periods per year.
- *NuvaRing* is a vaginal contraceptive ring containing a combination of synthetic estrogen and progestin hormones. The woman places the ring within the vagina and it remains there for three weeks. It is then removed for one week during which time the woman will experience her menstrual period.
- The *Contraceptive Patch* looks like a band-aid. A new patch is applied each week for three weeks and it slowly releases a combination of estrogen and progestin hormones through the skin.
- What is called, "The Morning After Pill," involves hormone doses about 2 to 5 times that of the traditional birth control pill. It works by either preventing ovulation and fertilization or in the event a pregnancy occurs, it renders the endometrium hostile, making implantation impossible (abortifacient). It is not known how the use of this procedure will affect the woman's return to fertility.
- This brief description provides limited information for women recovering from the use of these products. None of these methods is recommended by NWFS.

Though these contraceptives are not identical, the recovery from them is similar. For simplistic purposes, the contraceptives described will be referred to as "the Pill/Patch," unless one in particular is being referenced.

When thinking of the Pill/Patch one needs to consider a number of factors. First, there are several dozen types of pills including combined pills, progestin-only pills, and extended use pills. One must expect different responses to different types of pills. Second, some are predominantly synthetic estrogen or synthetic progestin. Since these are synthetic hormones, rather than naturally occurring ones, women charting while on the Pill/Patch cannot expect to see a typical cycle pattern. If the chart does appear typical, it is still reflecting the synthetic hormones and not a naturally occurring cycle. When a woman discontinues the Pill/Patch, she may notice one of the following patterns.

The most common occurrence is that typical cycles return right away, or within a cycle or two, after discontinuing the Pill/Patch. She may notice cycles that are longer than usual for her. She should not be misled by the artificial 28-day cycles experienced while on most pills and the Patch. Instead, she should recall her cycle pattern as it was before she took the Pill/Patch. There may be a very long delay before ovulation, sometimes months, and in rare situations, up to a year.

Certain information helps to assess the post-Pill/Patch phase. If this applies to you, ask the following questions. How long were your menstrual cycles before you took the Pill/Patch? How many years after your first menstrual period did you start the Pill/Patch? The menstrual cycle pattern takes 5 to 8 years to establish — this is known as the "adolescent" phase of your reproductive life. If you took the Pill or other hormonal contraceptives during this phase, the time it takes to re-establish your cycle pattern may be longer. How long did you take the Pill/Patch? What kind of hormonal contraceptive was it? What was its hormone content? In any case, charting your signs will help you understand what's happening. Discuss these factors with your NFP Provider.

Begin charting your temperature, tissue-paper, sensation, and cervix observations as you learn them. You will soon discover what is most helpful for your own situation.

What rules are recommended post-Pill/Patch recovery phase? The 6-5 Day Rule may be applied to the bleeding which occurs immediately upon discontinuing the Pill if the entire packet sequence was taken. As soon as a "Peak + temperature rise" occurs, apply the Sympto-Thermal Rule. For the following 4 to 6 cycles, it is best not to attempt to assume any pre-ovulatory infertility beyond Day 6. You need to learn your cycle pattern. If, after discontinuing the Pill/Patch, four weeks go by without a temperature rise, you may wish to apply the Basic Mucus Rule until you do see a temperature rise.

Since some women do experience a continuous discharge post-Pill/Patch, it is wise to chart the traits of the most fertile sign observed as well as the main symbol (Ø, M, EW-M). With this information, your NFP Provider can help you evaluate fertility even if a continuous discharge is present.

If your cycles are quite irregular with variable mucus, you may want to ask your healthcare provider about natural progesterone therapy to help your body "remember" how to cycle. This is a natural hormone supplement very different from the Pill/Patch's synthetic suppression of fertility. Administered properly, it can help the healing process. Additional information about natural progesterone can be found on page 66.

Post-Pill Cycle

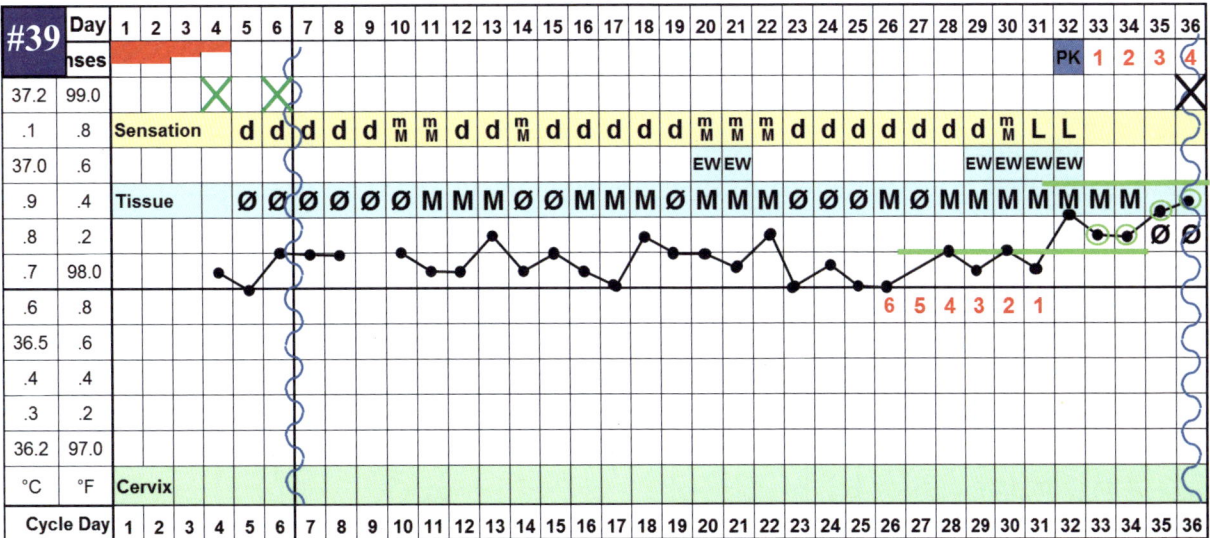

Stopping the monthly contraceptive pill mid-sequence may make returning fertility more confusing. In the long run, it may be easier to finish out the sequence and discontinue at that point. In order to avoid the potential abortifacient properties of the Pill, a couple can abstain from Days 10 to 20 of the "Pill Cycle." Once the woman has discontinued the Pill, the couple can begin applying the guidelines described on page 70.

Achieving pregnancy post-Pill/Patch. There is a higher incidence of miscarriage during the first six months after discontinuing the Pill. Since the mechanism is similar for the extended contraceptive pill and the contraceptive patch, it is assumed the following advice applies as well. For the couple desiring to achieve a pregnancy, it would be prudent to first allow the reproductive system ample time to return to a thoroughly normal state. The research of Dr. Erik Odeblad has shown that the woman's cervix ages an extra year for each year the Pill is taken; however, a pregnancy rejuvenates it by 2 to 3 years (http://www.woomb.org/omrrca/bulletin/vol25/no2/effects.shtml). If true menstruation doesn't occur within a year after discontinuing the Pill, be sure to consult your physician about it.

Injectables or "The Shot"

An injectable synthetic progestin such as *Lunelle* or *DepoProvera* are currently administered in 1 or 3 month intervals respectively. There is a two week "grace period" in which a woman can be late for the next shot of Depo-Provera (3 month version). The principle is the same as for the Pill/Patch. An absence of menstruation is common for the long-term injectable user; however, some women experience an increase in bleeding. In any event, the after effects are more long-lasting with Depo-Provera with longer delays in cycling.

Post-Injectable Cycle

When is a woman "post-injectable"? The post-injectable phase begins when the next shot is due. The actual return of fertility can be quite delayed. For example, the average return of menstrual cycles (not necessarily fertility) for women who are discontinuing *Depo-Provera* is ten months. Some women may experience an earlier return; however, others may experience a delay of one year or more in the return of their menstrual periods. The temperature level may be somewhat elevated during this transition because of the synthetic progesterone. The most common occurrence is prolonged dry days with a gradual return of cycling.

What rules are recommended post-injectables? The Basic Mucus Rule is recommended until the first Peak + temperature rise. Since it is common to experience intermittent spotting or bleeding during this phase, it is important to note that all bleeding other than true menses is to be treated as if it were EW-M. The only bleeding that is considered true menses is bleeding that occurs at the end of a sustained high temperature phase. Once cycling resumes, the Basic Mucus Rule should be discontinued. Then the couple should follow the Sympto-Thermal Rule and the 6-5 Day Rule for 4 to 6 cycles to learn the cycle pattern before applying further Relatively Infertile Time guidelines. If the woman observes only dry days, then the couple should apply a temperature-only rule to establish the Completely Infertile Time.

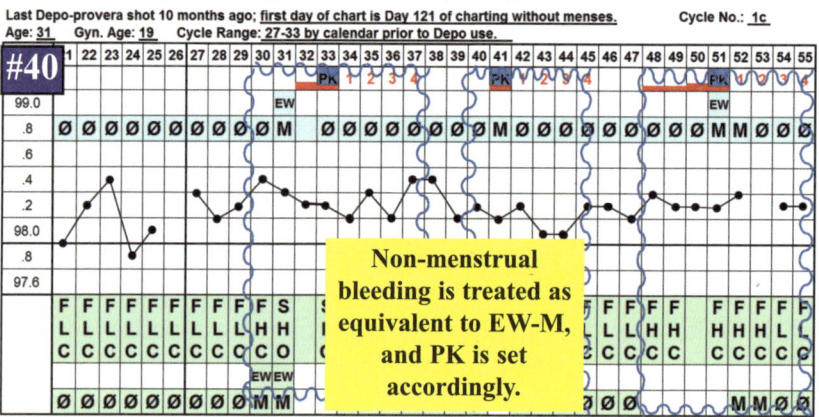

Non-menstrual bleeding is treated as equivalent to EW-M, and PK is set accordingly.

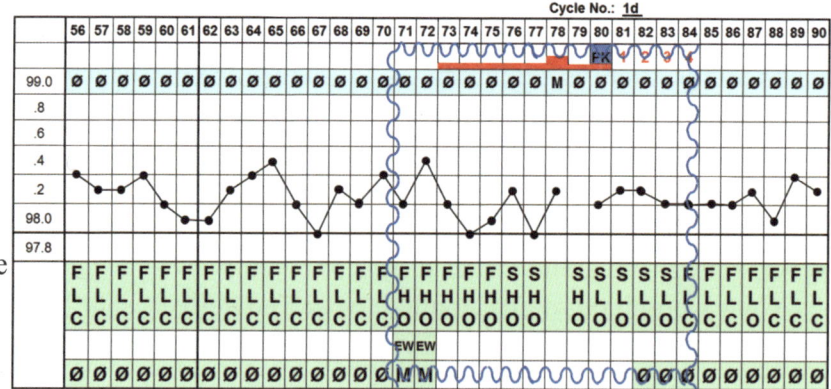

In Chart 40, after one month of observation the couple began applying the Basic Mucus Rule upon the recommendation of their NFP Provider.

Contraceptive Implants

The contraceptive implant, *Jadelle*, might be available for women. Implants are long-lasting contraceptives in the form of nonbiodegradable silicone rubber capsules containing steroid levonorgestrel. These contraceptive capsules are inserted into the woman's arm and slowly release synthetic hormones over a period of three to five years. The effectiveness gradually wears off over time. Excessive bleeding has been a common complaint and reason for discontinuation of *Norplant*.

When is a woman "post-implant"? The post-implant phase begins after the capsules have been removed or three to five years after insertion. The return to cycling is in general more rapid than with *Depo-Provera*.

What rules are recommended post-implants? The couple should follow the Sympto-Thermal Rule and the 6-5 Day Rule for 4 to 6 cycles to learn the cycle pattern before applying further Relatively Infertile Time guidelines. If the woman observes only dry days, then the couple should apply a temperature-only rule to establish the Completely Infertile Time. If, after discontinuing an implant, four weeks go by without a temperature rise, the Basic Mucus Rule is recommended until the first Peak + temperature rise. Once cycling resumes the Basic Mucus Rule should be discontinued.

Intrauterine Device (IUD)

Intrauterine devices (IUDs) are plastic devices which are inserted into the uterine environment. IUDs affect the sperm, ova, or the endometrium (as an abortifacient). There are two types of IUDs currently on the U.S. market: one containing copper and another type uses a synthetic progestin. Both act mechanically and chemically on the uterine environment.

The hormone-based IUD is supposed to be removed and replaced annually (Progestasert) as the hormonal component diminishes during that time. The copper-based IUD needs to be replaced every 8 to 10 years.

What is "post IUD"?

Once the woman has the IUD removed she is post-IUD. What rules are recommended post-IUD? Cycling generally returns quickly post-IUD. The Sympto-Thermal Rule (STR) is recommended unless there is no Peak + temperature rise by four weeks after the removal of the IUD. In that case, the couple should follow the Basic Mucus Rule. Once cycling resumes, the Basic Mucus Rule should be discontinued. Whenever cycling resumes, the STR and the 6-5 Day Rule are recommended for 4 to 6 cycles to learn the cycle pattern before applying further RIT guidelines. If the woman observes only dry days, then the couple should apply a temperature-only rule.

The above guidelines are general. Couples should consult with an NFP Provider to learn the most effective guidelines to apply in their individual situation.

After Childbirth

After you have a baby, many things in your life change and you make lots of adjustments. Whether you breastfeed or not, your menstrual cycles will return, but the process may be delayed. Some women experience bleeding before they have a return to ovulation. For example, a woman can ovulate and be fertile even before her menstrual periods return. Some women have become pregnant between babies but not had a menstrual period between the two deliveries.

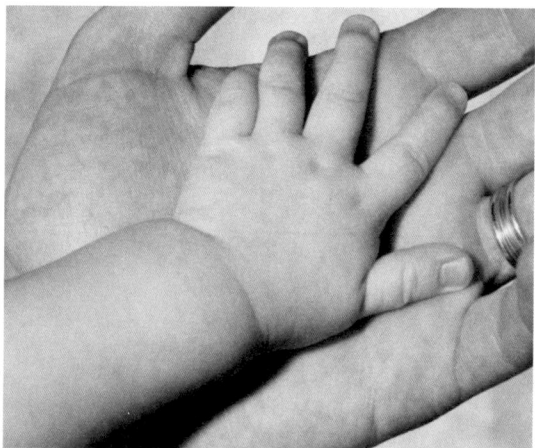

How will you know when fertility returns? Cervical mucus signs will precede ovulation, and a sustained temperature rise will accompany it, so you need to chart your cervical mucus and temperature signs.

There is typically a transition time before your cycles will return to what you experienced before pregnancy.

The Transition Time — the first two or three cycles you may experience:
- Long episodes of mucus, which may come and go without a subsequent temperature rise.
- Spotting or even full bleeding that is not true menstruation. You can identify non-menstrual bleeding because it isn't preceded by a biphasic temperature pattern.
- The first temperature rise may be somewhat shallow, less obvious than usual.
- The first high-temperature phase may be somewhat shorter than usual, perhaps less than eight days.
- Determine with your healthcare provider when it is medically safe for you to resume intercourse after childbirth. Dr. Roetzer says that intercourse is usually medically safe beginning the 4th week after delivery; it mainly depends on how the woman feels.
- If you are avoiding pregnancy, follow the Basic Mucus Rule, (see page 53).
- Once the conditions of the Sympto-Thermal Rule (STR) are met, the bleeding afterward can be considered true menstruation and the 6-5 Day Rule applied.

After this initial time of transition, your cycles should return to what is normal for you. Perspective is always helpful, so patience, cooperation, and a sense of humor really help. Check regularly with your NFP Provider for further clarification of your circumstance.

Miscarriage

A miscarriage is the naturally occurring early loss of a pregnancy. It is often an emotionally traumatic experience. Estimates are that between 15 percent and 30 percent of all pregnancies end in miscarriage. The risk of miscarriage increases with age, with the highest proportion occurring in women between 35-44 years. There are a variety of reasons. During the first trimester, the reasons are usually related to abnormalities in the development of the baby or genetic defects. During the second trimester, the most common reason is an incompetent cervix. Third trimester losses are properly called stillbirth.

If miscarriage occurs or you experience any unusual pelvic pain or vaginal bleeding, consult your healthcare provider at once. Early intervention can, in some instances, save the baby's life. If the miscarriage can't be stopped, remember that anyone can baptize in emergency situations.

The time after miscarriage can be emotionally upsetting for both husband and wife. Many people try to deny the loss of their unborn child and fail to grieve the loss. Couples have found that there is some comfort in knowing the why. Sometimes women feel guilty wondering if they did something to cause the miscarriage. It might help to remember that almost all miscarriages occur because of an abnormality. You didn't cause it. Remembering this child is important to heal your loss. Some parents name their unborn child. There are a number of books and pamphlets which address the loss of a pregnancy. If you are feeling sad or depressed after experiencing a miscarriage (even if it has been some time), be sure to seek professional help – you are not alone. Check with your NFP Provider for local resources.

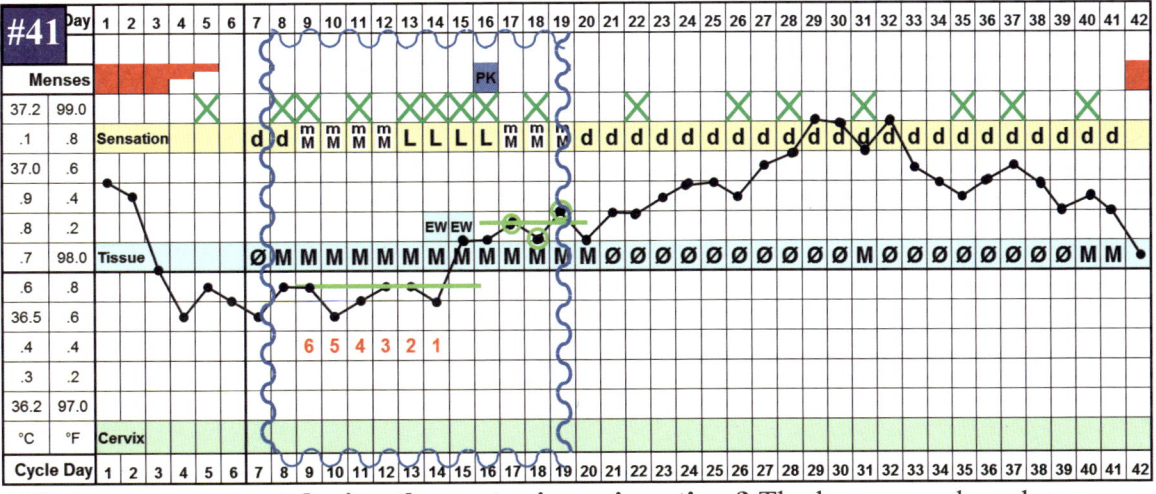

What can you expect during the post-miscarriage time? The longer you have been pregnant, the more the time after miscarriage will be like the time after childbirth. Some physicians consider it medically safe to try to achieve pregnancy again immediately after a miscarriage, while others recommend the woman experience at least one normal menstrual period first. You should check with your physician first.

Fertility can return as soon as two to four weeks after miscarriage and most often by eight weeks. If you wish to avoid pregnancy at this time, abstain from all genital contact and intercourse until the Sympto-Thermal Rule is met.

After Childbirth When Not Breastfeeding

Women who are not breastfeeding at all will most likely have their first true menstrual period at about six to twelve weeks after childbirth, but occasionally it may be a little earlier or later.

How do you practice NFP during this time? Begin charting temperature and cervical mucus signs at three weeks after delivery or as soon as the discharge is gone.

If four to six weeks go by without a temperature rise, you may wish to apply the Basic Mucus Rule until you do see a temperature rise.

As soon as "Peak + temperature rise" occurs, apply the Sympto-Thermal Rule. The experienced NFP user can then resume the instructions followed before the pregnancy. The recommendation for the new user is to follow the 6-5 Day Rule until a typical cycling pattern resumes. Establishing infertile days beyond Day 5 or 6 usually takes 4 to 6 cycles of experience and should be discussed with your NFP Provider.

Breastfeeding

Women who breastfeed their newborn children may notice several months go by before their first menstrual period after childbirth. Some women who nurse for a lengthy time may also notice an extended time without menstruation lasting up to two years or more. But there is no cause for alarm. Nature is providing an extended time of natural infertility to care for the child. The suckling of the child causes the woman's body to secrete a hormone, prolactin. It is known that prolactin inhibits ovulation.

Benefits to Breastfeeding
- Prolonged time of natural infertility.
- Beneficial to the child's immune system.
- Assists in mother-child bonding.
- Women who breastfeed experience greater bone density and fewer hip fractures in menopausal years.
- It may be a protective factor with some subtypes of breast cancer.
- It's convenient and inexpensive.

One cannot, however, assume that as long as a woman breastfeeds her child she will experience infertility. The kind of breastfeeding that causes this extended time without menstrual periods after childbirth is intensive breastfeeding.

"Intensive Breastfeeding" means that the baby's nourishment comes totally and exclusively from sufficient suckling by the baby at the breast and...
- There are no supplements. Use of a breast pump or manually expressing milk does not always suppress the return of fertility the same way "intensive breastfeeding" does. It makes a difference.
- Nursing is distributed evenly throughout the 24-hour day, with eight to ten feedings daily and with the baby's longest interval between two feedings to be no more than eight hours.
- If one were to add up the total nursing time, there should be a minimum of about two hours total of nursing each day.

Intensive breastfeeding as defined above will certainly provide twelve weeks of infertility after childbirth, and in most cases more. But with any departure from intensive breastfeeding, fertility may return earlier. For example, if the baby nurses fewer than eight times daily or sleeps longer than eight hours, but is otherwise "intensively breastfeeding," then fertility may return sooner than 12 weeks after childbirth. On the other hand, even after supplements start, infertility might continue.

It is the recommendation of Northwest Family Services, whether or not you are intensively breastfeeding, to begin charting at least the cervical mucus sign once the postpartum discharge is complete (or at least between six to eight weeks postpartum). If you chart the cervix, it may take from 6 to 12 weeks for it to return to its normal condition, so you may want to delay this observation during this time.

Taking occasional temperature readings to verify the overall low level is also helpful. It is not uncommon, however, during the early months after childbirth, before cycling resumes, to see an erratic temperature pattern. The primary emphasis should be on the cervical mucus.

Below is the chart of a woman who is intensively breastfeeding; it begins at 8½ weeks after childbirth:

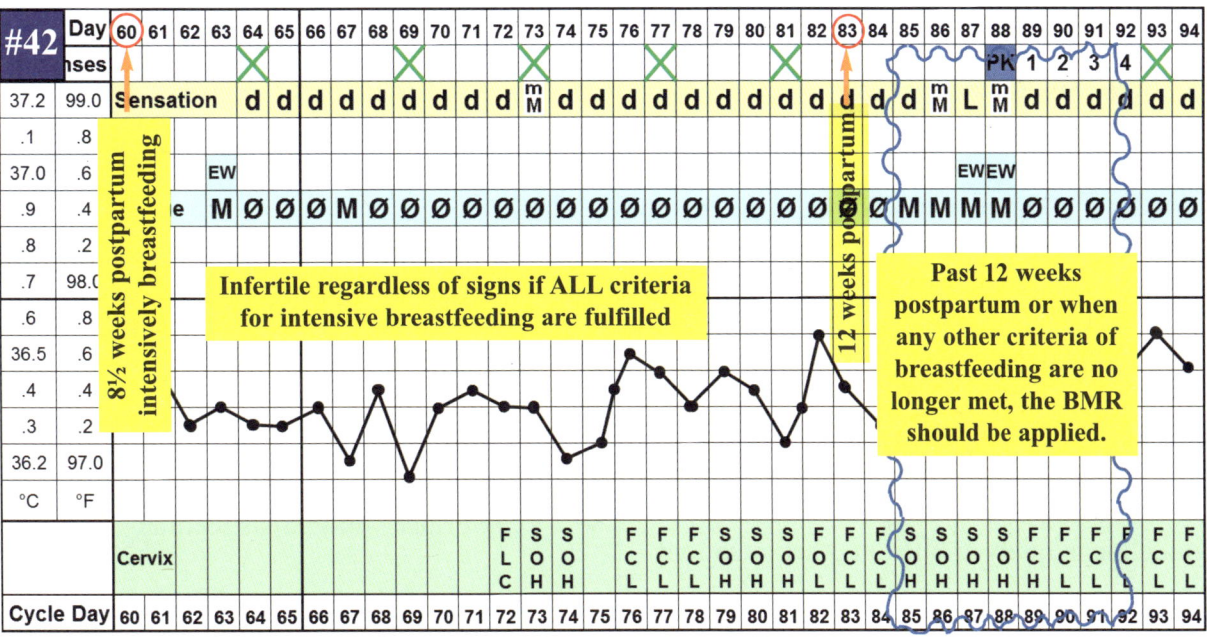

After 12 weeks postpartum if you are intensively breastfeeding, or as soon as you establish a pattern if you are not intensively breastfeeding, begin to apply the Basic Mucus Rule, page 53. Once you experience a "Peak + temperature rise," apply the Sympto-Thermal Rule.

Breastfeeding and NFP

During the extended infertility after childbirth, there are three basic patterns:
- Continuous dryness.
- Continuous moistness or mucus.
- A mixture of mucus days and dry days.

To assume infertility you need to identify your own basic unchanging pattern. An unchanging pattern means the ovaries are at rest, not yet preparing for ovulation. Some women, not realizing this, or mistakenly expecting a cycling pattern, become anxious when there is "never any mucus" or when there is "mucus, but it never changes." Yet that is just what they are looking for to identify infertility. The day-to-day sameness indicates a lack of ovarian activity. Once the hormone levels begin to rise, there will be a change in the mucus pattern.

It takes a few weeks of observation to determine what the basic pattern is if it's something other than continuous dryness.

Whenever cervical mucus occurs, you will need to chart its traits (e.g., color, amount, stretch, tissue glide, how often observed during the day, and sensation). It is fairly common for a breastfeeding woman to experience a continuous moist sensation. Check with your NFP Provider as it may be possible to treat as a consistent, unchanging pattern.

Some women find the firm, low, closed cervix as added confirmation of infertility during the unchanging external cervical mucus symptom.

What if you notice patches of mucus? Some breastfeeding women notice dry days punctuated on and off by "patches" of one or two days of sticky mucus or moist sensation. This makes applying the Basic Mucus Rule (BMR) very restrictive. There is a special adaptation of the BMR called the "Patch Rule" which can be used effectively while breastfeeding until cycling resumes. This guideline is rarely applied in other situations.

Lactational Amenorrhea Method (LAM)

LAM is a method of family planning based on extensive evaluation of breastfeeding women around the world. When the following conditions are met, breastfeeding alone is 98 percent effective during the first six months after childbirth:
- No bleeding after 56 days postpartum.
- Fully or near fully breastfeeding.

This application needs to be discussed with your NFP Provider

Patch Rule

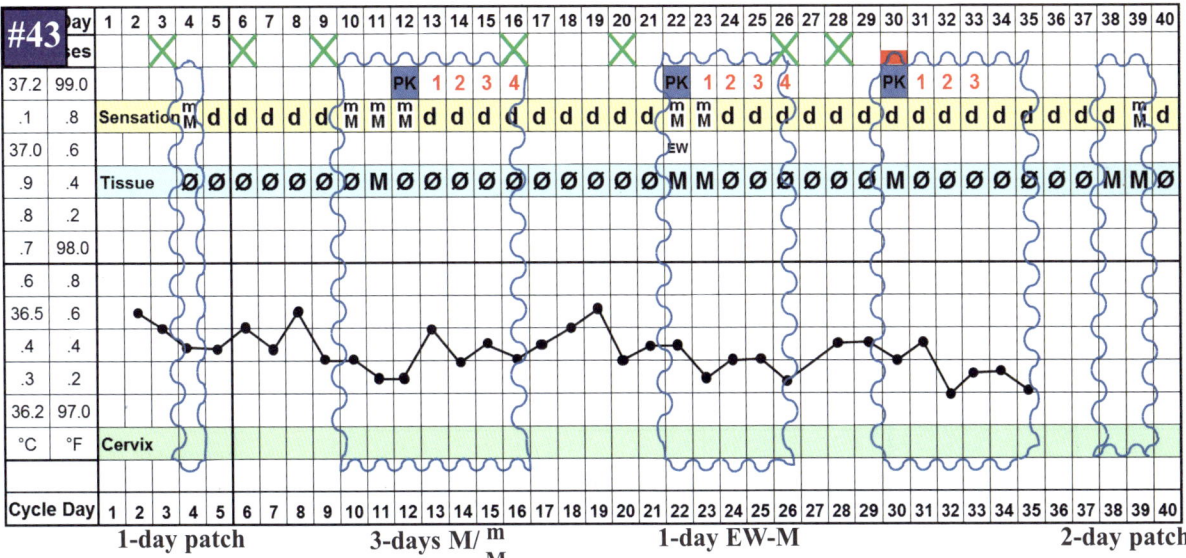

The guidelines are as follows:

- Apply a Pk + 4 count to every episode of L, EW-M, non-menstrual bleeding, and to all episodes of three or more days of **M** or $\frac{m}{M}$.
- Any one- or two-day "patch" of **M** or $\frac{m}{M}$ is considered fertile, but no Pk + 4 count is required afterward.
- Consult with your NFP Provider on the application of this guideline.

Applying the Basic Mucus Rule to a pattern of dryness is fairly easy, but applying it to a pattern of continuous **M** or $\frac{m}{M}$ or a pattern of cervical mucus and Ø days requires the advice of your NFP Provider. Your NFP Provider can help you evaluate your chart and find appropriate rules to follow until cycling resumes. There are advanced guidelines not discussed in this manual.

Return to cycling. When "Peak + temperature rise" occurs, apply the Sympto-Thermal Rule and the 6-5 Day Rule for a few cycles. Because some women may experience erratic temperature swings during breastfeeding, continue to observe for cervical mucus for the first cycle or two. If cervical mucus returns and the temperature drops, assume fertility and call your NFP Provider. Once cycling resumes, an experienced user of NFP may decide to follow the guidelines she used prior to pregnancy.

The actual transition from not-yet-cycling to cycling often coincides with the weaning process and may require, during the two or three cycles of transition, a longer period of abstinence than will be normal during typical cycling. Here is the completion of the first cycle after childbirth for the woman whose early postpartum chart was shown earlier:

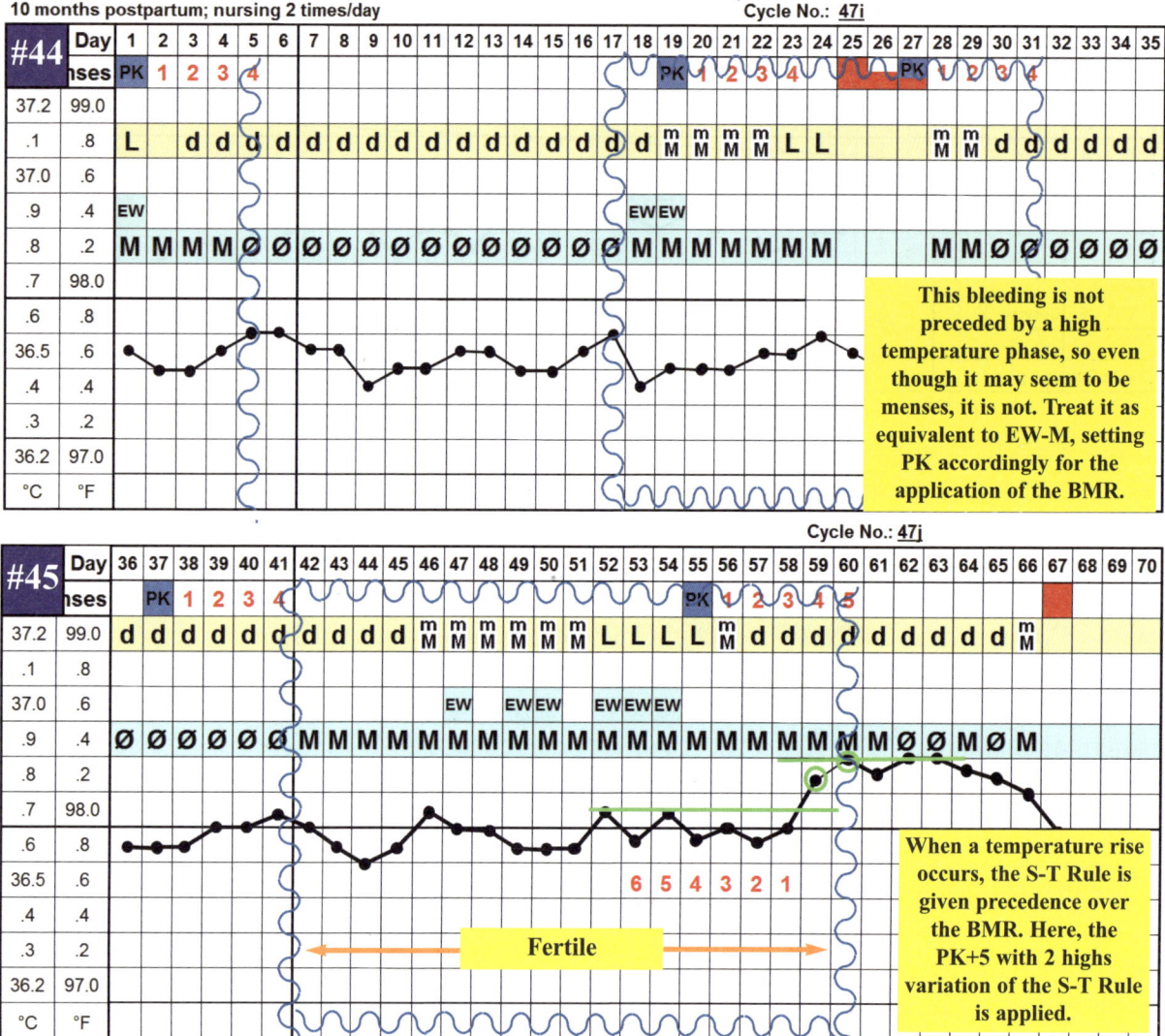

Return of Fertility during Breastfeeding

When your menstrual periods resume, it is not unusual to notice a short high-temperature phase for the first two or three cycles: In Chart 45, the high-temperature phase was only 8 days; the next cycle was 35 days long with an 8-day high-temperature phase; after that the cycles were typical and easy to understand. There are as many cycle patterns as there are women, but the charts above illustrate what some women may experience as their cycles resume after childbirth. It can be a difficult time, but it is not impossible. It is best dealt with by patient cooperation and humor between the spouses and the skilled assistance of your NFP Provider.

During the extended pre-ovulatory phase after childbirth, the mucus signs and cervical changes are your anchor point for determining infertility and possible fertility. Some advocate NOT taking temperature at all during breastfeeding, and consider it an unnecessary bother.

There are several reasons why others may choose to take the temperature. There may be several or even many cervical mucus episodes, each reflecting hormonal fluctuations but not ovulation. The absence of a temperature rise confirms that you are still in the pre-ovulatory phase; even just checking periodically and finding that the temperatures are still low assures you that you're not pregnant.

There may also be bleeding from time to time due to hormonal fluctuations. The bleeding needs to be treated as if fertile, like EW-M, unless it's true menstruation; bleeding is considered to be true menstruation ONLY if preceded by a high-temperature phase in which the Sympto-Thermal Rule or temperature-only rule was fulfilled.

When you do see "Peak + temperature rise," you know you are infertile for the rest of the cycle and can expect a menstrual period in a week or two if you abstained from all genital contact and intercourse during the fertile time.

Finally, if you DON'T take your temperature, but DO become pregnant, you won't know when pregnancy occurred. Some couples use breastfeeding for child spacing, particularly if for them the delay in cycling is lengthy. They may choose to achieve pregnancy even before the woman's first true menstrual period. The recorded temperature rise indicates which cervical mucus episode was associated with ovulation, and the continued high-temperature phase of 18-20 days or more indicates that pregnancy has occurred. The due date is based on the Peak Day and initial temperature rise as the approximate date of conception.

Other important points. In some respects, while breastfeeding, you are truly "eating for two." It is generally best to continue with prenatal vitamins. Pay attention to a well-balanced eating regimen. If you are attempting to lose weight after childbirth, consult with your healthcare provider on a proper diet for breastfeeding mothers.

If you have questions or concerns about breastfeeding, contact the local LaLeche League or a lactation consultant for excellent support and concrete advice.

There is a normal time of sexual readjustment following childbirth. It is not uncommon for women to experience vaginal "dryness." Husbands can be attentive to tender foreplay to overcome this. Fatigue and a general 24-hour-a-day disruptive schedule also contribute to the "lack of interest" which some women experience after giving birth. Make time for rest and to be alone with each other even if only for short intervals of time.

Premenopause

Once a woman over age 40 has failed to menstruate for 12-14 months, she is considered to be in menopause. There is a timespan of several years (usually five to eight years) gradually leading up to menopause, called premenopause or peri-menopause. If ovarian function stops before age 40, it is considered "Premature Ovarian Failure," and cycling may resume or be experienced sporadically. The age when menopause is usually experienced is between 45 and 55 years old. During this time the menstrual cycle may become sporadically longer or shorter than before. The typical cervical mucus and temperature patterns may begin to change. Non-menstrual bleeding occurs more frequently and may be longer and heavier than a menstrual period. This type of bleeding is easily identified because no temperature rise occurs before or after it. Charting your signs will help provide an accurate record of what is happening.

Overall fertility declines dramatically after age 40. This means that couples desiring to achieve a pregnancy can expect it may take some time or that they may be unsuccessful or that a pregnancy will more likely end in miscarriage. This may be true even if the woman has a typical cycle pattern with a biphasic temperature rise and a changing cervical mucus pattern.

Premenopause and the short cycle. It is more common for couples to want to avoid pregnancy during this transition time of their life. NFP can be successfully and effectively used during the premenopause years. One of the first signs of premenopause may be an unexpected short cycle. On the other hand, women may experience longer cycles, and couples avoiding a pregnancy will more frequently apply the Basic Mucus Rule instead of waiting for a temperature rise, if they wish to avoid extended abstinence. Observing for a temperature rise confirms that ovulation has occurred. As long as possible, it is advisable to follow the Sympto-Thermal Rule.

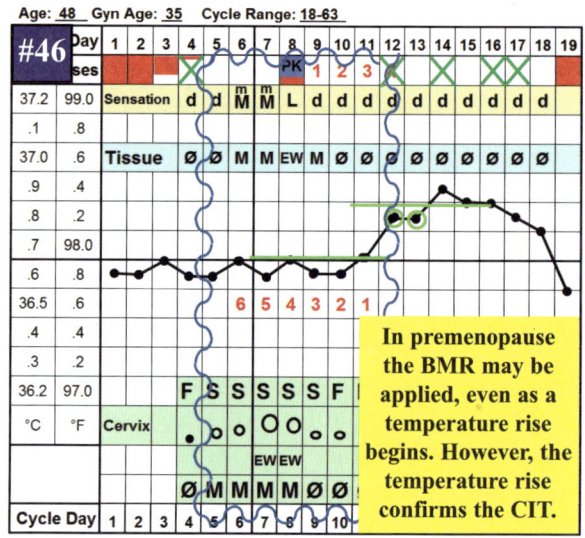

Less Cervical Mucus.

During premenopause some women notice a marked decrease in the amount or quality of mucus by tissue-paper check and sensation. This can occur as early as the late thirties and early forties, even before the woman is in premenopause. Chart 47 is an example in which the

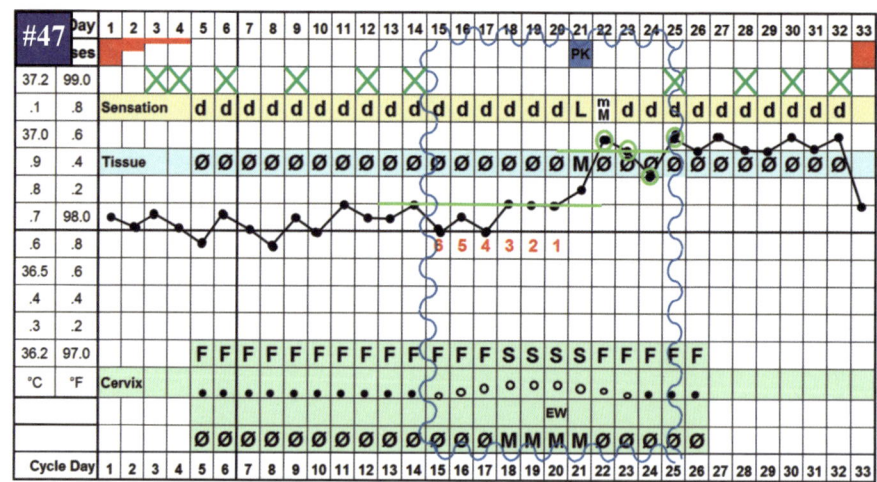

woman noticed dryness by tissue and sensation, but had symptoms by the cervix signs. In such a case, Peak Day is set by the mucus found at the cervix (see Day 21).

The Cervix can help. Take care to assess all bleeding correctly, and report any unusual bleeding to your physician at once. The temperature pattern will distinguish true menstruation from any unusual bleeding. The cervical exam may be especially helpful at this time.

The temperature is important when evaluating a long cycle. A continued low-temperature phase assures you that you are indeed NOT pregnant, even though it may have been a long time since your last menstrual period, and even though there may have been several episodes of mucus or bleeding or both since then. Premenstrual spotting tends to occur more frequently after age 35. When it does, Day 1 = the first day of bright red bleeding or the first day the temperature returns to or below the Pre-Rise Baseline and stays there — whichever comes first. Chart 48 illustrates application of the Basic Mucus Rule and the Sympto-Thermal Rule in a long 74-day premenopausal cycle:

Premenopause and NFP

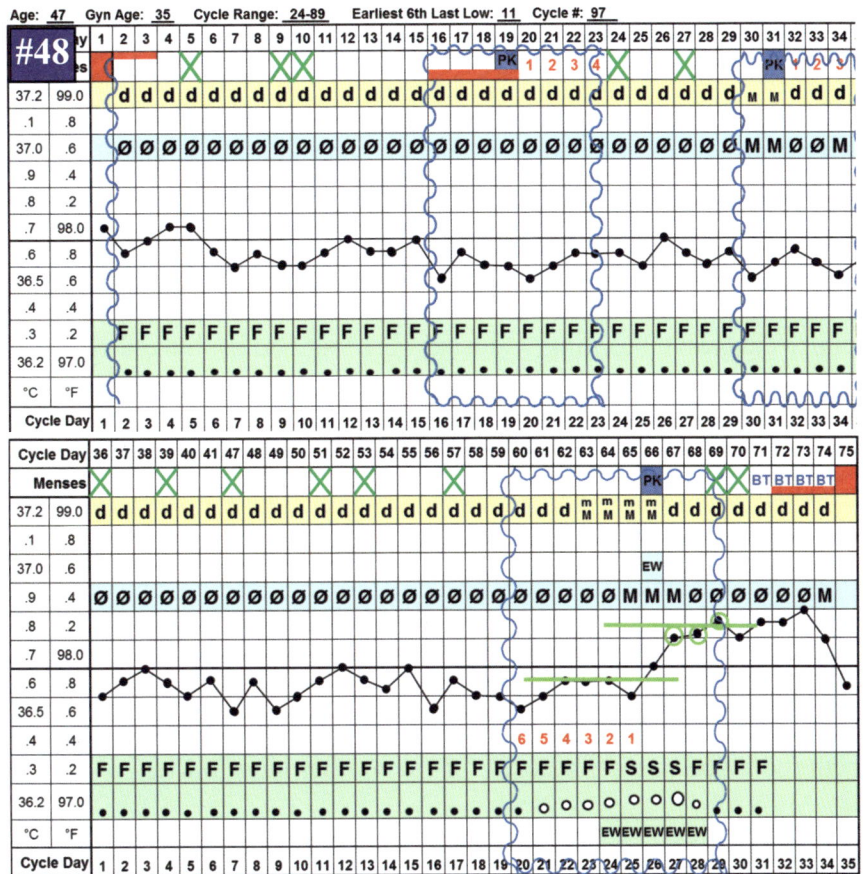

All bleeding other than true menstruation is considered fertile, and is treated as if cervical mucus. Non-menstrual bleeding is equivalent to EW-M and L for purposes of setting Peak Day. Apply the Basic Mucus Rule to episodes of non-menstrual bleeding. When the temperature rise occurred in the chart above, the Sympto-Thermal Rule was applied as usual.

Other symptoms which accompany premenopause are as follows: We strongly recommend reading *Fertility, Cycles, and Nutrition* by Marilyn Shannon and *What Your Doctor May Not Tell You About Menopause* by Dr. John R. Lee for his thorough discussion of the benefits of natural progesterone as well as other healthful remedies.

Hot Flashes: They are experienced as a sudden sensation of intense heat which occurs throughout the body, especially in the face and neck area. Hot flashes or flushes usually last only a minute or two and may be accompanied by excessive perspiration followed by chills or shivers. Some women experience night sweats. Hot flashes occur because the body's thermostat setting is narrowed and minor temperature changes trigger an exaggerated response. They occur in response to fluctuating hormone levels.

Consult a health care provider for medication or a naturopathic doctor for a natural remedy.

Vaginal Dryness: As the estrogen levels decrease, the vaginal walls become thinner and there are fewer secretions, sometimes resulting in painful intercourse. Non-hormonal lubricants or greater attention to foreplay may reduce these symptoms. Vitamin A is said to aid with this condition. Continued intercourse helps tissue flexibility. In severe cases, an estrogen vaginal cream is necessary.

Weight Gain: A part of aging is an increased tendency for a slower metabolism. Attention to one's eating habits and a regular exercise program such as walking, swimming or other aerobic activity, amounting to a minimum of 30-60 minutes per day, helps tremendously. Stretching along with weight-bearing exercises are particularly good in maintaining flexibility and preventing bone loss.

Fatigue: Women who experience excessive bleeding, insomnia, and general body changes are understandably going to be fatigued. Vitex, magnesium, and chlorophyll (source of Vitamin K) may help reduce excessive bleeding. Unusual bleeding and prolonged fatigue should always be evaluated by a healthcare provider. Prudence signals a need for extra rest, attention to one's eating habits and exercise routine, and a re-evaluation of one's activities and priorities.

Osteoporosis: Much controversy surrounds the issue of osteoporosis ("increased bone porosity" resulting in brittle bones). This malady is associated with the time after menopause rather than with premenopause itself. Recent evidence demonstrates that the risk associated with hormone replacement treatment exceeds its benefits for most women who use it continuously. Alternative therapies include moderate weight bearing exercise, Vitamin D, calcium, magnesium, and sodium fluoride. This would need to be evaluated with one's health care provider. A benefit of breastfeeding children earlier in life is that it increases bone density with a subsequent reduction in hip fractures for the mother later in life.

Note: Hormone replacement therapy or a combination of estrogen-progestin replacement therapy may affect the woman's cycle, making charting and interpretation confusing or impossible.

CHAPTER SIX: COMMON QUESTIONS

Few factors interrupt the fertility cycle. There are some treatments which can impact the symptoms. The following are responses to some of the most frequent fertility-related questions.

Premenstrual Syndrome (PMS). PMS occurs during the 1-2 weeks of high temperature before menstruation, and is distinct from "dysmenorrhea" (painful menstruation), which occurs during the one to two days before menstruation or during menstruation.

Dysmenorrhea can be treated successfully with prescription or non-prescription anti-prostaglandins (ibuprofen is an anti-prostaglandin). Magnesium supplements have been shown to reduce severe menstrual cramps. Sometimes birth control pills are prescribed for dysmenorrhea, but ibuprofen products and magnesium are specific to the symptoms, only need to be taken a few days each cycle as needed, and are non-hormonal.

PMS has been categorized into four main groups by Guy Abraham, M.D. He formulated a vitamin-mineral regimen which reduces or alleviates the following symptoms (Optimox Corporation, http://www.optimox.com, 800-223-1601):

- *Anxiety PMS*: nervous tension, irritability, mood swings.
- *Cravings and Carbohydrate Intolerance PMS*: especially chocolate is craved, followed a few hours after ingestion by headaches, palpitation, fatigue, and the "shakes."
- *Weight Gain PMS*: water retention, swelling of the face, hands, and feet, abdominal bloating, and breast tenderness.
- *Depression PMS*: withdrawal, confusion, crying, insomnia, and forgetfulness.

PMS takes several forms, and its incidence and severity seem to increase with childbirth, age, stress, poor diet, and lack of exercise. The NFP chart provides an awareness of one's symptoms over several cycles and aids in accurate diagnosis of PMS. Vitamin, mineral (especially magnesium), and other supplements such as Evening Primrose Oil help many women in reducing PMS. Vitex has been shown to significantly reduce PMS symptoms as has natural progesterone cream.

A severe form of PMS is known as premenstrual dysphoric disorder (PMDD). Symptoms associated with PMDD include depression, anxiety, irritability, anger, and other symptoms occurring exclusively during the two weeks preceding menses. PMDD is a severely distressing and disabling condition and treatment is available. Check with your healthcare provider if you are noticing these symptoms as there are effective treatments.

Perimenopausal Symptoms. The debate over hormone replacement therapy (HRT) has been settled. A landmark study published in the *Journal of American Medical Association*, July 17, 2002, stirred a major firestorm as it revealed that women on estrogen-progestin replacement therapy were at increased risk for several cancers particularly those women who were using the treatment for 10 or more years. Women using HRT also experienced an increased risk of blood clots, strokes, and heart attacks. Physicians are no longer routinely prescribing HRT for women over age 40. Women are advised to consult their healthcare providers for direction on the matter.

The FDA panel concluded that since HRT products contain low levels of hormones, it must be assumed that the higher dose contraceptives products, e.g., birth control pills, contraceptive patch, could have similar effects.

See the "Premenopause" section on pages 82-84 for further recommendations.

Toxic Shock Syndrome (TSS). The Food and Drug Administration advises regarding TSS and tampons:

- Women can almost entirely avoid risk of TSS by not using tampons. The diaphragm, contraceptive sponge, and cervical cap have been associated with increased risk of TSS. There are no reported cases of TSS associated with the *NuvaRing* as of this printing.
- Women can reduce their risk of developing TSS by cutting back on their use of tampons during menstruation. For example, wear tampons during the day, and sanitary napkins on light flow days and in the evening. Researchers have found that continuous use of tampons does increase the risk of TSS.
- Women with any symptoms of TSS while using a tampon should remove it immediately and contact a doctor at once. The symptoms of TSS are sudden high fever (102°F [38.9°C] or higher), vomiting, and diarrhea. Other symptoms that may be noticed include dizziness, sudden drop in blood pressure, a rash that looks like a sunburn, severe muscle ache, bloodshot eyes, or a sore throat. TSS can be successfully treated with prompt medical care.

Oral and Genital Herpes or Genital Warts. Care should be taken during observation not to spread oral herpes (HSV1) to the genital area, and particularly to the cervix, or genital herpes (HSV2) to the oral area. The same is true of human papilloma virus (HPV), commonly known as genital warts, which is highly contagious. Spreading these viruses can be minimized by washing one's hands properly before and after observation, and, when genital herpes is active or genital warts are present, to refrain from checking the cervix. Intercourse during outbreaks of genital herpes or genital warts should be avoided — seek medical advice as there are treatments available. The data does not indicate that the use of condoms will reduce the transmission of genital herpes or HPV.[8] Women infected with HPV should seek regular gynecological examinations as certain strains of this virus are associated with an increased risk of cervical cancer.

---

8. Centers for Disease Control, "Male Latex Condoms and Sexually Transmitted Diseases," July 2009, http://www.cdc.gov/nchstp/od/latex.htm, http://www.medinstitute.org/.

Fertility awareness enables a woman to be attentive to early health needs which require medical intervention. This is a special benefit of NFP. In addition, good health care practices require regular gynecological examinations including a Pap exam and breast examination. These routine procedures save lives. All women should routinely examine their own breasts as a preventive measure for breast cancer (see page 95). A special reminder note is placed on the NFP chart. While there are women who are at greater risk for breast cancer, such as women who have a family history of breast cancer or women who have had an abortion, there are significant numbers of women who develop breast cancer each year and there is no known risk associated. It is best to examine the breasts during the early part of the cycle as some women experience tender and even lumpy breasts during the high-temperature phase.

Cycle Irregularity. While some women naturally have long or erratic cycles, a medical evaluation may be in order to rule out new or chronic conditions. Thyroid deficiencies can cause non-typical cycles. If your Pre-Rise Baseline is usually on or below 97.0°F (36.2°C), investigate this possibility. Ovarian cysts often result in erratic cycles. Being underweight or overweight can contribute to erratic cycles. Transitioning from childbirth, breast-feeding, post-hormonal treatment, or the adolescent gynecological phase are times associated with longer cycles. Stress can lengthen the cycle too.

Some remedies include progesterone therapy. It may be prescribed during premenopause or when there is cycle "irregularity" which mimics a corpus luteum: the progesterone inhibits ovulation and induces a high-temperature phase. One may continue as usual to apply the Sympto-Thermal Rule and the Relatively Infertile Time rules one has been using, as advised by her NFP Provider. Natural treatments include natural progesterone cream and Vitex agnus castus which have been associated with regulating the cycle (consult a nutritionist or herbal specialist).

Medications and Cervical Mucus. Always chart any medication taken. Either the medication or the condition for which it is being taken or both may be relevant. But even though there are potential side effects, a given woman may not experience any impact on the menstrual cycle. Here are a few general recommendations:

Antihypertensives containing a diuretic may decrease mucus (wait and see). *Vitamins* reportedly help to increase mucus (especially B-complex and A). Vitamin B_6 may suppress prolactin and is a note of caution for breastfeeding women. Megadoses of vitamin C may decrease mucus. *Minerals* can also be an aid to fertility. Magnesium supplements can result in shorter menstrual periods, and shorter and clearer cervical mucus patterns, as well as reducing excessive bleeding. Magnesium may also reduce the "morning sickness" some women experience during early pregnancy.

With any medication or condition that contraindicates pregnancy, a couple is advised to restrict intercourse to the Completely Infertile Time. For example, both vaccination against measles, rubella shot, and Accutane (isotretinoin), an anti-acne preparation, are associated with birth defects if administered while the woman is pregnant.

Current Medical Research
FACT SHEET: Drugs Which Affect the Cervical Mucus, by Hanna Klaus, M.D.

Drug	Usually Prescribed For	Site of Effect	Type of Effect
Acetylcystene (mucomist)	Asthma, Cystic fibrosis	Local	If sufficiently absorbed, could increase or thin mucus.
Alpha Antitrypsin	Cystic fibrosis	Local	Could increase or thin mucus.
Ampicillin	Infections	Local	Could increase or thin mucus.
Antidepressants, Antipsychotic: e.g., Thorazine, Mellaril, Triavil, Parnate, Valium, Prozac, MAO (Monoamino Oxidase) Inhibitors	Depression	Local and systematic	A variety of menstrual disturbances ranging from menorrhagia to menopause have at times been reported with Prozac (PDR 1991).
Antihistamines	Cold, cough, allergies	Local	Can decrease amount of mucus, can cause thickening or dryness.
Antitumor drugs: e.g., Busulfan, Cyclophos-phamide, Cytotoxic agents, Mercaptopurine, Chlorambucil, Actinomycin	Used to treat tumors. (Actinomycin is also used for systemic fungus infection.)	Systemic	Suppress ovulation, induces menopausal (high) levels FSH, LH.
Atropine	Antispasmodic	Local	Can decrease amount of mucus, can cause thickening or dryness.
Belladonna	Antispasmodic	Local	Can decrease amount of mucus, can cause thickening or dryness.

This fact sheet was prepared for the DDP for NFP, NCCB, by Hanna Klaus, M.D., NFP Center of Washington, D.C. Inc., with the kind assistance of Sr. Paulette Elking, Ph.D., 1993, 1999.

Drug	Usually Prescribed For	Site of Effect	Type of Effect
Buserelin	Antigonadotropin used to treat endometriosis, etc.	Hypothalamus	A variety of menstrual disturbances ranging from menorrhagia to menopause could occur.
Cimetidine (Tagamet)	Used to treat peptic ulcers.	Local and systemic at level of hypothalamus or above.	A variety of menstrual disturbances ranging from menorrhagia to menopause could occur. Inhibits histamine, also pituitary gonadotropins.
Clomiphene	Ovulation Induction. Antiestrogen drug.	Systemic	Reduces or suppresses mucus. A variety of menstrual disturbances ranging from menorrhagia to menopause could occur.
Cough mixtures with Antihistamines, i.e. Phenylephrine	Cough	Local	Can decrease amount of mucus, can cause thickening or dryness.
Danazol	Antigonadotropin, used to treat endometriosis, etc.	Systemic	A variety of menstrual disturbances ranging from menorrhagia to menopause could occur.
Dicyclomine	Antispasmodic	Local	Can decrease amount of mucus, can cause thickening or dryness.
Estrogens	Ovulatory dysfunction	Local and systemic	Produces mucus with fertile signs; may also produce strong cholinergic action, i.e., may cause dryness whether local or systemic.
Guafenesin	Expectorant found in cough syrups	Local	Could increase or thin mucus.
Leuprolide	Antigonadotropin, used in treatment of endometriosis, etc.	Systemic	A variety of menstrual disturbances ranging from menorrhagia to menopause could occur.

Drug	Usually Prescribed For	Site of Effect	Type of Effect
Oral contraceptives	Contraception	Local and systemic	Produce sticky, yellow, or white opaque mucus (progressive effect).
Potassium Iodide	Expectorant found in cough syrups	Local	Could increase or thin mucus.
Progesterones	Ovulatory dysfunction	Local and pituitary	Produce sticky, yellow, or opaque mucus.
Propantheline	Antispasmodic	Local	Can decrease amount of mucus, can cause thickening or dryness.
Tamoxifen	Used to treat breast cancer.	Systemic	Antiestrogen, reduces or suppresses mucus. A variety of menstrual disturbances ranging from menorrhagia to menopause could occur.
Urecholine (Bethanechol)	Cholinergic agent - urinary retention	Local and systemic	Theoretically could thin secretions.

Miscellaneous Notes
- Vitamin B_6 may suppress Prolactin, a caution to nursing mothers. Some think that B complex vitamins increases cervical mucus.
- Any increase in exercise or any rapid change in weight may suppress ovulation.
- Fabric softener, and tampons may increase or distort recognition of mucus.
- Smoking – *active and passive* – has been associated with high nicotine and cotinine levels in cervical mucus, which in turn are associated with dysplasia. No observable physical change has been reported.
- *One More Soul* (http://www.omsoul.com/) provides a directory of NFP-only physicians.

Nutrition Tips & Self Care for Hormonal Imbalances (Excepted from NWFS brchure)

1) Love your Liver.

What does your liver do? It detoxifies drugs, chemicals and poisons. It produces bile and stores vitamins. Most importantly, it breaks down and gets rid of excess hormones. The liver converts estradiol, an active form of estrogen, into estriol, a safer form of the hormone. High estrogen has been associated with an increased risk of endometriosis. So, loving your liver helps lower the active form of estrogen to help fight endometriosis.

You can protect the liver cells by providing the nutrients it needs with a balanced diet. The nutrients the liver needs to stay healthy are anti-oxidants (Vitamin C, E and Selenium,) and beta-carotene. These nutrients can be found in seeds, nuts, berries, and other fruits.

You can improve bile flow by eating more bitters. Foods that are bitter include: dandelion leaf and root, endive, radicchio, mustard greens, and beet greens.

You can improve detoxification by eating foods that contain sulphur compounds. Some sulphur-containing food are garlic, dandelion, cabbage, and brussel sprouts.

Eating ground flax seeds daily can also help the liver bind the excess estrogen and get rid of it. Flax seeds contain lignans which bind to the extra estrogen. Flax seeds are also a stool softener and can help prevent constipation.

2) Promote Regular Bowel Movements.

The liver does all this work to convert estrogen into a safer form and then it leaves the body through the feces. If you don't have a regular bowel movement, your body could take back that extra estrogen.

You can help your body with regular bowel movements by eating things with fiber. Foods high in fiber include vegetables (e.g., asparagus, broccoli, carrots, collard greens) and grains (e.g., bran, barley.)

3) Improve the Immune System.

When endometriosis is occurring, the immune system sends macrophages to go to tissues to clean up the debris caused by infection or inflammation. A build-up of these macrophages can prevent fertilization of the egg, increase the rate of adhesion formation, and increase inflammation, causing more pain. Increasing the flow of lymph can help prevent macrophages from sitting in the uterine cavity.

Castor oil packs daily to your pelvic area increases the flow of lymph. A castor oil pack is made by putting 2 tablespoon of the oil on a piece of flannel. Apply it directly to the lower abdominal area, with a towel on top, and a heat pack atop for 30 to 40 minutes daily.

4) Provide precursors for estrogen and progesterone.

Eating 2 tablespoons of ground flax seeds or pumpkin seeds the first 14 days of your cycle (Day 1 of your cycle is the first day of bright red bleeding) and taking 2 tablespoons of fish oil provides essential fatty acids that are needed for the estrogen hormones in the first half of the cycle. Eating 2 tablespoons of ground sunflower seeds or sesame seeds and 2 tablespoons of evening primrose oil or borage oil provides essential fatty acids for the progesterone hormones from day 14 of your cycle until the first day of your next period. Starting this rotation can help your body establish and maintain a better ratio of progesterone to estrogen.

5) Eat an Anti-Inflammatory Diet.

Foods can contain chemicals that promote inflammation. Some inflammation is good, but having too much is bad. Too much of these inflammation-aiding chemicals can cause more uterine muscle spasm and dilate blood vessels, increasing blood loss and pain. Eating more Omega 3 foods (e.g., fish) promotes anti-inflammatory chemicals.

6) Regular exercise.

Regular exercise decreases the rate of estrogen production.

CHAPTER SEVEN: BACKGROUND INFORMATION

Hormones

The external bodily signs observed with NFP reflect internal hormonal changes during the menstrual cycle. During the first part of the cycle, the follicle (the housing around the egg) begins to grow. The follicle produces estrogen. Rising estrogen levels cause the cervix to become softer, higher, more open, and "wet" with changed, increased, and flowing cervical mucus. There is a change in the vaginal sensation to moistness (^m_M) or lubrication (L). And Sticky Mucus or Egg-White Mucus is noticed on the toilet tissue paper.

In the process of releasing the egg, the follicle changes into what is called a "corpus luteum" (yellow body) while remaining in the ovary. It continues to secrete estrogen but now also produces progesterone. Progesterone is designed by nature to assist eventual pregnancy: it prevents a further ovulation, enriches the uterine lining, forms a thick mucus plug at the cervix to keep out bacteria, and causes the waking temperature to rise and stay higher. The cervix becomes distinctly firm, low, and closed again, like at no other time in the cycle.

Pregnancy occurs at conception when the sperm fertilizes the egg cell in the upper third of the fallopian tube. It takes about one week for the tiny new human being to travel down the fallopian tube and to implant in the uterus. At this point the new life hormonally signals the corpus luteum to keep on functioning and thereby continues its own life by blocking the occurrence of menstruation.

The corpus luteum will wait about two weeks after ovulation for "word" of pregnancy. If a "message" is not received by the time implantation would have been completed and the pregnancy successfully under way, it stops functioning. When the corpus luteum stops producing estrogen and progesterone, the uterine lining loses its support, and the result is a menstrual period, at about two weeks after ovulation. Due to the drop in progesterone, there is also a drop in the waking temperature back to the low level.

Ruth Taylor, M.D., speaks of the concept of the "Symphony of the Menstrual Cycle" in which she relates the menstrual cycle to a score of a symphony.[9]

Each instrument must come in on cue and perform in harmony so that the result is a beautiful symphonic masterpiece.

So it is with a woman's menstrual cycle. Body functions need to be in harmony just as the musical instruments in an orchestra. Each body function works precisely so that ovulation, the main event of the menstrual cycle, will take place.

The conductor of this symphony is the pituitary gland, which stimulates the ovary to release its hormones. The ovarian hormones, in turn, influence all the other functions (instruments) in the menstrual cycle.

After estrogen peaks and rapidly falls, LH (luteinizing hormone) from the pituitary gland spikes — like the clash of cymbals — and triggers ovulation. The egg bursts forth from the

---

9. Gallagher, A., Heinzen, A., Hogan, R., Taylor, R., Teaching Catholic Family Values, Leaflet Missal Inc., 1996.

ovary. The egg will live no longer than one day if it is not fertilized.

After ovulation, the corpus luteum is formed from the empty follicle and secretes progesterone. Progesterone causes a quieting of the uterus as the glands of the endometrium fill with nutrients which would nourish the tiny baby. Progesterone also causes the woman's body to become a little warmer, as demonstrated by the rise in the temperature after ovulation.

The cervical mucus during most of the cycle is dense and thick and remains in the cervix. With the rise of estrogen, the mucus changes; at this time, the cervix produces a normal, healthy discharge which the woman is aware of around the time of ovulation at the vaginal opening.

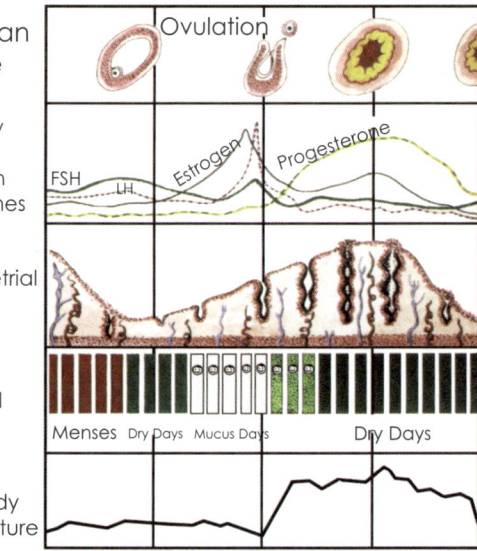

With every normal menstrual cycle, an ovum (egg) matures and is ovulated (released). At the same time, the uterus is prepared to receive a new life if conception takes place. If not, the cycle repeats itself, like the theme of a symphony, over and over during the woman's reproductive life. Non-menstrual bleeding can be pathological bleeding, implantation spotting, ovulation bleeding, or bleeding due to fluctuations in hormones such as after childbirth, during premenopause, or in some cases of stress.

Ordinarily, women can easily tell whether or not the bleeding is the menstrual period, but sometimes there can be confusion. If you are charting temperature, there is rarely a problem identifying menstrual bleeding. You know that the only bleeding which is true menstruation is the bleeding that comes at the end of a high temperature phase. All bleeding other than true menstruation is considered fertile.

Menstrual Cycle Myths...

Unfortunately there are still quite a few myths about the menstrual cycle and NFP that need to be put to rest:

The "normal" 28-day cycle. This is an average, approximately true for a whole population of women, but most individual cycles are longer or shorter.

"Mid-cycle" ovulation. Ovulation occurs about two weeks before the following menstruation, regardless of cycle length. It is only "midcycle" if the cycle happens to be about 28 days.

Cycle Myths
- The "normal" 28-day cycle.
- "Mid-cycle" ovulation.
- "Random" ovulation.
- "Induced" ovulation.
- "Old" sperm and eggs causing miscarriages and disabilities.

"Random" ovulation. Once ovulation occurs, further ovulation is suppressed. The "random ovulation" myth is partly traceable to the mental habit of dating ovulation in relation to the previous menstrual period, and misunderstanding references to this variable preovulatory time: e.g., "I was told I can ovulate on any day of my cycle," which was misunderstood as "it can happen anytime even more than once a cycle."

"Induced" ovulation. In rabbits intercourse can bring on ovulation, but not in humans. The egg cell must grow through a specific developing process before ovulation can occur. This developmental process is precisely why NFP works.

"Old" sperm and eggs causing miscarriage and disability. This theory was based on very questionable transfer of laboratory animal data to humans in non-laboratory settings, or of very poor, very small surveys, in genetically unique populations, to the population at large, etc. All relevant studies reveal that there is absolutely no basis for this theory.

Breast Self-Exam

Breast cancer sometimes strikes indiscriminately. Being attentive to the fertility cycle should cue women more easily into doing regular breast self-exams. It truly can save one's life. The NFP chart is marked with a breast exam reminder on cycle Day 6. The best time of the cycle to do a breast self-exam is during the Relatively Infertile Time, because the breasts can naturally become sore and even lumpy during the high-temperature phase.

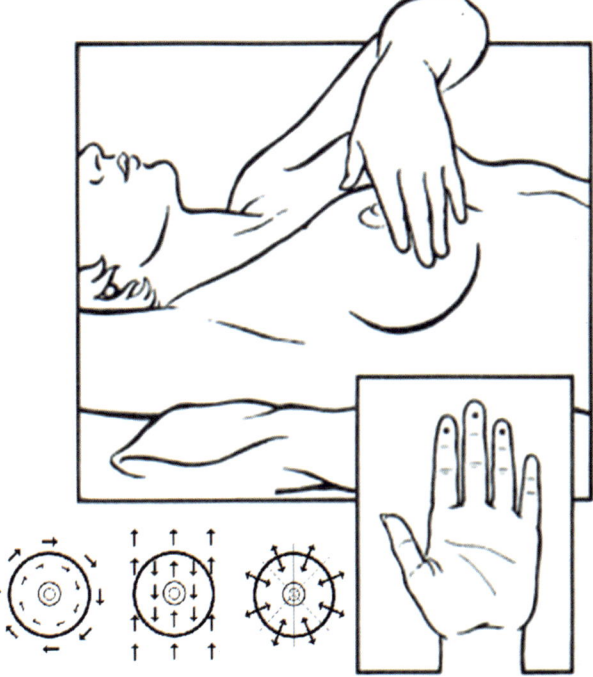

Women should conduct a visual observation of the breasts before a mirror observing for changes in contour or discoloration of the skin or changes in the nipple.

The self-exam also involves manual observation of the breasts as shown in the picture on the right following the pattern displayed. A detailed description is available from the American Cancer Society.

In the event breast cancer is discovered, there is evidence that the timing of the surgery with respect to the menstrual cycle can improve the survival rate. "In 1991, a report in Lancet confirmed previous findings that timing of surgery influenced breast cancer survival. Women with node-positive premenopausal disease who had surgery during the luteal phase were found to have up to 30 percent better survival than women who had surgery in the late follicular phase" [the Relatively Infertile Time].[10]

---

10. Harlow, S., Ephross, S., "Epidemiology of Menstruation and Its Relevance to Women's Health," *Epidemiologic Review*, vol. 17, no. 2, 1995.

Effectiveness

How effective is NFP? It depends. Do you want to achieve pregnancy? Or to avoid? Or are you ambivalent? In any case the single most important factor for "effective" Natural Family Planning is the cooperative effort between husband and wife to follow all the rules for observation, charting, and chart interpretation.

If you are capable of achieving pregnancy, fertility awareness skills enable you to know the days when you are possibly, or even probably, fertile. But procreation is a complex process involving many factors. There is no guarantee that use of even the apparently most fertile days will result in pregnancy. The couple experiencing difficulty in achieving a pregnancy can feel frustration, a reminder to us that fertility is a gift, not an automatic fact that can be taken for granted.

Avoiding pregnancy involves abstaining from any genital contact when the rules of NFP indicate possible fertility. To be "99 percent effective" a rule can be wrong no more than once in a hundred years, that is, no more than once in over a thousand cycles, or over a year for a hundred couples.

Completely Infertile Time. The Sympto-Thermal Rule, the Mean Temperature Rule, and the BBT Rule are 99.9+ percent effective. These figures come from over 40 years of experience with over two hundred thousand charts observed in the Austrian physician Josef Roetzer's research.

Relatively Infertile Time. All of the following guidelines yield a 99+ percent reliability —the 6-5-0 Day Rule; the Earliest 6th Last Low Rule crosschecked against tissue, sensation, and cervix; use of the tissue and sensation dry days after menstruation when crosschecked with a firm, closed, and dry cervix; and dry days after menstruation if a moist sensation regularly precedes the first sign of cervical mucus on the tissue.

A couple with normal fertility must expect to become pregnant within a very few cycles when intercourse occurs on days when cervical mucus is present (especially EW-M days or the first day or two after Peak).

NFP studies generally show the Sympto-Thermal Method to have a 99+ percent method effectiveness and about 90-98 percent use effectiveness,[11] which takes into account misunderstanding, carelessness in charting, and chance-taking. During regular cycles, when a Mucus-Only Method is used, the method effectiveness runs about 99+ percent, and the use effectiveness is about 85-97 percent.[12] Calendar Rhythm has a use effectiveness rate of about 75 percent. Statistics, however, can be confusing. Standard Days Method, which target women who may benefit has an 80% typical use effectiveness.[13] Occasionally, popular magazines will lump together the effectiveness figures for NFP, including Calendar Rhythm, without making a clear distinction between the different approaches. The language used by family planning professionals also includes terms such as "perfect use" and "imperfect user." These are technical terms. Perfect use means the couple uses the method exactly according to instructions, consistently and correctly every time. For example, perfect use is generally reported for condom effectiveness, even though, like NFP, it is a behavior-dependent method. The terms incorporated in this book are lay terms.

---

11. The European Natural Family Study Groups. "European Multicentre Study of Natural Family Planning (1989-1995): Efficacy and Drop-Out." Advances in *Contraception*, 1999, 15: 69-83.
12. Hilgers, T. W., et al, *Journal of Reproductive Medicine*, 1998, 43:495-502.
13. Research-to-Practice -- Standard Days Method. (n.d.). Retrieved 07 28, 2009, from *Institute for Reproductive Health*: http://irh.org/RTP-SDM.htm

"Use effectiveness" figures from various studies are not always easy to compare. One must pay attention to how each study defines its categories of pregnancy. In "real life" highly motivated couples using the Sympto-Thermal Method can expect a 99 percent effectiveness from the use of NFP.

Motivation is one of the most important factors for NFP effectiveness, assuming that sound rules have been taught and are properly understood. In all forms of family planning, NFP included, limiters have a much lower pregnancy rate than spacers.

"Spacers" are couples who say they're postponing a desired pregnancy for the time being — but desire to conceive during a given future timespan beyond that set by the study design.

"Limiters" are couples who enter a study stating that they wish to have no more children at all — or at least do not intend to conceive during a given future timespan set by the study design questionnaires they receive.

"Limiters" tend to be more serious about learning and following the guidelines for avoiding pregnancy, whereas "spacers" tend to be more careless about it and sometimes have not discussed their family planning intention with each other.

The majority of "unintended" pregnancies are due to behavior rather than biology. That is, the couple becomes pregnant while knowingly using a fertile day as opposed to experiencing a pregnancy from intercourse on a day the method indicated was infertile. This is not unexpected. The rules of the various modern NFP methods have been carefully developed to cover the range of conditions under which intercourse may lead to pregnancy. Even so, no type of family planning in use (natural or artificial — including surgical sterilization) is 100 percent effective for avoiding pregnancy. There are the rare, but real, "surprise" or "method" pregnancies that occur when the NFP instructions for avoiding pregnancy are correctly understood and followed. But an "unplanned" (or "unintended" or "unforeseen") occurrence of pregnancy does not mean an "unwanted" (or "unaccepted" or "unloved") child.

Couples experiencing what they believe is a true "surprise pregnancy" should contact their NFP Provider at once. The chart may advance the knowledge about the conditions under which pregnancy can occur — future couples will benefit. And, in any case, the consultation will provide personal moral support.

Some couples wonder if it would be "more effective" to use contraceptives rather than abstinence during the fertile time. Not necessarily, nor would it be NFP. First, the contraceptives are entirely unnecessary for avoiding pregnancy during most of the cycle because the couple is infertile anyway. Second, abstinence never leads to pregnancy; contraceptive intercourse may. Barrier contraceptives are said to "work best" only when used consistently and with spermicides that will alter the cervical mucus observation, making accurate interpretations difficult. It makes no sense to discover the fertile time and then use barriers at the only time they can fail, nor does it make sense for a couple to cause uncertainty about where they are in the cycle and increase dependency on the barrier contraceptives.

Apart from all that, much of the interpersonal dialogue and growth that can occur, when periodic abstinence is followed, is lost or diminished.

Ongoing data collection from Northwest Family Services clients has shown that those who fail to complete the instructional series, take chances with barrier contraceptives at the fertile time, or otherwise second-guess the rules to see if they really mean what they say have a higher unintended pregnancy rate than those who complete the series, abstain while fertile, and follow instructions as given. In one formal study, the "limiters" had no pregnancies at all.

The Historical Foundations for NFP

The above pages stand on the shoulders of researchers and couples from all parts of the world and many decades of experience. And what you learn about NFP makes you part of that worldwide experience.

Some elements of NFP observation and interpretation have long been a part of other, non-Western cultures: e.g., an awareness of the soft, high, open, wet cervix as the best time for conception is part of the tradition among the women in some parts of Africa. What is being discovered today, from a Western perspective, is how God from the beginning has equipped us with a body language for understanding fertility and for entering into dialogue with him and each other about his creative intentions for us.

Calendar Rhythm was born with the independent discoveries by Knaus (Austria, 1929) and Ogino (Japan, 1923) that ovulation occurs at a relatively constant time *before* menstruation (but at a quite variable time after the start of the cycle). Calendar Rhythm had to calculate the fertile time based on the range in the lengths of previous cycles. But it would gradually be supplanted by a discovery of the day-to-day signs that accompany the fertile and infertile times, regardless of past cycle history.

Temperature Methods were developed in the 1930's onward to determine post-ovulatory infertility. This made it unnecessary to use a calendar calculation for the onset of the Completely Infertile Time. A German priest, Fr. Wilhelm Hillebrand in 1929 developed for his parishioners the first practical methodology. Dr. Rudolf Vollman (1930's on) developed the "Mean BBT Rule"; Jan Holt (1950's), the "3 higher than 6" concept. Dr. Gerd Döring (1950's) developed the "Earliest 6th Last Low Rule" as an extension of the use of the temperature. This provides a more individualized approach to setting a borderline for the end of the pre-ovulatory infertile time. Dr. Josef Roetzer has since promoted a "modified" Döring Rule, with a crosscheck for cervical mucus against the earliest previously recorded 7th Last Low. In 1967 the World Health Organization adopted, in committee, the "World Health Organization BBT Rule."

Cervical Mucus and its changes had been described in the mid-1800s in France. Its relation to fertility was known by gynecologists, but this knowledge was for a long time never translated into an educational process to teach its observation and interpretation. It was Dr. Josef Roetzer (1951) who first formulated a "Sympto-Thermal Rule": he made the interpretation of the temperature rise *dependent* upon the cessation of the cervical mucus. Dr. Josef Roetzer first developed the tissue-paper exam (published 1965) utilizing an "open and fold" procedure for checking mucus. His system also incorporates an awareness of sensations (especially the sensation of "moistness" that is experienced as "up inside, from within" the vagina, as well as sensations experienced "at the lips" of the vagina). Drs. John and Evelyn Billings (from 1954 on) researched in NFP; by 1973 they had developed a "mucus-only" method which they called the "Ovulation Method." They developed the first methodology to use the mucus symptom at the vaginal entrance (especially emphasizing sensations at the vaginal entrance, and the Basic Mucus Rule), as a guide for all circumstances, for both infertile and fertile days, without use of temperature as a crosscheck. Dr. Thomas Hilgers (1978 on) developed a mucus-only methodology relying only upon tissue-paper exam with "finger test" for mucus, called *FertilityCare*™ Method (previously known as "The Creighton Model").

Checking the cervix for mucus and cervical changes was popularized already in the late 1940's by Dr. Edward F. Keefe. Developing more refined rules for the cervical exam and integrating these into educational programs was largely the work of John and Sheila Kippley of the Couple to Couple League, SERENA of Canada, and Dr. Josef Roetzer.

High-Tech NFP. Type in "ovulation detection devices" on your favorite Internet search engine and any number of sites will display their wares. Litmus tests, hormone tests, cervical mucus assessments, computerized devices, and interpretative software packages are all available for NFP users. The Marquette Method (MM) uses the Clear Blue Easy Fertility Monitor combined with NFP fertility observations. Those couples using MM who were taught by trained NFP Providers experienced a 97-98 percent effectiveness rate.[14] There is a big difference between identifying the event of ovulation and accurately predicting the beginning and end of the fertile time. Some women appreciate double checking their charting information with a technological device. As of this printing, there are no products that *consistently* provide the information a couple needs to avoid a pregnancy at the same effectiveness level that the modern NFP methods provide.

We will leave it up to the reader to research the various products. Recall, however, the adage, "Buyer Beware." Before pursuing "new and improved" NFP approaches discuss the efficacy of the product with your NFP Provider.

---

14. Marquette University. (2004). Efficacy of the Marquette Method of Natural Family Planning. Retrieved July 28, 2009, from *Marquette Natural Family Planning*: http://nfp.marquette.edu/efficacy.php

Test Your Knowledge

1. What is the most important factor in getting a good temperature record?

2. You should do the tissue exam (select one):
   a) at least four times per day.
   b) after you go to the bathroom.
   c) before and after you go to the bathroom, every time.

3. If you can't lift any mucus off the tissue, but you felt the tissue glide when you wiped, how would the observation be charted?

4. How much mucus you see is more important than the kind of mucus you see. True or False

5. Which signs are crosschecked to establish Peak Day?

6. How do you find the six last lows?

7. Where do you draw the Pre-Rise Baseline (PRB)?

8. How much higher than the Pre-Rise Base is the Full Thermal Shift Level drawn?

9. For temperatures to count toward the fulfillment of the Sympto-Thermal Rule, two criteria must be met. What are they?

10. When does infertility begin according to the Sympto-Thermal Rule?

11. Before assuming infertility beyond the 6-5 Day Rule, you should look for a consistent pattern, comparing the first sign of fertility with the location of...

12. Couples who absolutely must avoid a pregnancy should...

13. If a woman's cycle seems to be affected by stress, should a couple alter the rules they are applying for pregnancy avoidance? Yes or No

14. When a woman's cycling pattern changes, the couple should continue to apply the same rules, just doing so very carefully. True or False

15. The BMR is applicable in non-cycling situations or in situations where the woman has a long RIT. True or False

16. If a woman's mucus pattern is disturbed, a temperature-only rule can be applied. True or False

17. If a couple has a hard time interpreting the woman's pattern, they should (check all that apply):
    a) abstain until the pattern stabilizes
    b) call their NFP Provider for advice
    c) assume they are infertile since fertility would show a clear pattern.

18. Barrier methods of contraception can confidently be used during the method-defined fertile time. True or False

19. How many high temperatures indicate pregnancy?

20. Do mucus and cervix observations help identify pregnancy? If so, how...

21. A couple wanting to achieve pregnancy should focus intercourse during which days of the cycle?

22. A woman can learn to pinpoint the day of ovulation after she uses NFP for several months. True or False

---

Answers:
1. Consistency, see page 18.
2. c.
3. EW-M.
4. F.
5. Tissue and sensation.
6. See page 44.
7. See page 34.
8. 0.4°F [0.2°C].
9. Above the PRB and after Pk Day, see page 33.
10. See page 33.
11. Sixth last low temperature.
12. Restrict intercourse to the CIT.
13. See page 40.
14. F (check with their NFP Provider).
15. T.
16. T.
17. b.
18. F.
19. 18-20 high temperatures identifies pregnancy.
20. No, but the mucus and cervix signs do help identify the best time to try to achieve a pregnancy.
21. PFT, see page 61.
22. F (she can only identify the Possibly Fertile Time).

CHAPTER EIGHT: LIVING WITH NATURAL FAMILY PLANNING

Natural Family Planning — "Natural"?

Some claim that periodic abstinence is "unnatural," even though it is not surgically, mechanically, or chemically invasive. Yet NFP does presume that we are humans, not mere creatures of instinct. It takes for granted that we are capable of rational decisions and self-control in the expression of sexual feelings, and unselfish love for others.

Some would suggest that NFP is "unnatural" because it is not "easy" — it requires thought and some effort. Of course if one defines "natural" as what is "easy," "spontaneous," or "impulsive," then NFP could be said to be "unnatural." But isn't that kind of "natural" merely a definition of what is usually called irresponsible or immature?

> "NFP was something I thought we should do, but didn't necessarily want to. I knew it had some hard lessons to teach me." Mike Fuller

Wouldn't it be more consistent to think about sexuality the way we do about other aspects of life? We respect as normal the desire to excel, to understand, to enhance, and to develop instead of taking "the easy way out." When we view the grace of a dancer or the drama of the gymnast or the dexterity of the professional basketball player, don't their movements appear easy, spontaneous, even natural? Yet the skill which they display is gained through a commitment to self-discipline. So the fact that NFP takes effort, understanding, and principled decision-making does not make it any the less "natural." On the contrary, it leads one to believe that NFP is natural — an avenue to human fulfillment rather than an obstacle to it.

In reality the details of NFP methodology soon become routine, "second nature." But that's natural too. For we are creatures of habit, and the good habits that are developed are called "virtues," that is, character strengths or abilities to accomplish effortlessly what has become "second nature" to us by acquired practice. For instance, a thoroughly truthful person "spontaneously" tells the truth, but someone used to lying as a way of coping with mismanaged responsibility may find honesty "unnaturally difficult." So too, the sexual mastery in NFP is a challenge to discover a truly human kind of "spontaneity" in sex and marriage that may seem difficult at the beginning, as another pattern is being abandoned. Mother Teresa of Calcutta defined NFP as "self-control out of love." It highlights how the "No" to sex of periodic abstinence is part of the "Yes" to one's spouse and family — an expression of real love.

From Fertility Awareness To Fertility Acceptance

Basically there are two elements to NFP: first, learning to observe, chart, and interpret the cycle signs; and then, deciding to have sexual intercourse or abstain during the fertile time. After the initial enthusiasm of learning fertility awareness wears off, the couple faces the challenge of fertility acceptance. Part of fertility acceptance is the recognition that fertility is a normal and healthful part of the human person, as is sexual expression that is right ordered and within the context of a loving marriage. Periodic abstinence, an integral part of NFP, needs to be integrated within the life of marriage and family life.

Difficulties may crop up when husband and wife disagree about their family planning intention or are ambivalent about whether or not to have a child now. NFP challenges the couple to come to terms, honestly, with their real family planning intention and how they feel about themselves as parents or future parents. This is an ongoing process, and it requires soul searching and mutual support of husband and wife for each other.

Periodic abstinence is not always easy for a couple. But "easy" is a relative term. A person with a diabetic condition may find it hard to abstain from sweets, but a good reason to do so — health — can make even a difficult thing livable. The same is true for NFP. It is natural to experience tension with periodic abstinence: sometimes the tension will be greater and at others barely noticed. Some couples maintain perspective by reminding themselves of why they are abstaining and why they have chosen to use NFP. Some couples find it helpful to formulate on paper their own unexamined feelings about the matter. What are our reasons for avoiding, rather than attempting a pregnancy? For using NFP, rather than something else?

When abstinence is difficult or motivation to continue to chart lessens, couples sometimes discover, to their surprise, that they really have no good reason to further postpone pregnancy and in fact desire another child. On the other hand, they might discover that they really do want to avoid pregnancy but other factors seem to be at work: Is the woman looking for support and interest in charting from her husband? Have they just not bothered to continue strengthening their relationship in non-genital ways?

Positive Aspects Of Periodic Abstinence

A person's sexuality encompasses many dimensions beyond one's gender. True, it is one's gender: male or female. Yet men experience life in a masculine way that is only predominantly, but not exclusively, male, and women experience life in a feminine way that is only predominantly, but not exclusively female. The differences between men and women embrace the psychological and spiritual as well as the physical. And the differences serve not to isolate the two sexes, but to call them forth from within themselves to find their fullness in each other in friendship.

According to psychologist Carl Jung there is an anima or feminine component in each man's personality, and an animus or masculine component in each woman's personality. Each must come to know and accept that component of the other within himself or herself in order to be psychologically and spiritually healthy. Some see in sexual attraction a spiritual dimension: it is Adam's eternal search for completion in Eve, his missing rib, and her search for completion in him as well. Sexual attraction manifests its primordial meaning as one of drawing us out from within ourselves and leading us to interact with others (it is said to engender feelings of compassion and tenderness for others). Sexuality is by nature not turned in upon self. It is at root a search for unity and human intimacy with others. Becoming aware of the longing for male-female partnership helps to understand that attraction is not merely a genital response but a need for interpersonal friendship. Rollo May summed this up well: "[F]or human beings the more powerful need is not for sex, per se, but for relationships, intimacy, acceptance, and affirmation."

Sexual expression is thus a form of touching meant to imprint a closeness and unity on the mind and heart of the couple. This bonding goes beyond the mere experience of physical sensations in intercourse — the sensations without the marital bonding are but a counterfeit of true sexuality. And it involves more than procreation — even though the search for unity finds a special, endearing and enduring, incarnation in the child of their love.

The bonding requires a fundamental and total regard for one's spouse as a whole person, with a mind, a soul, a heart, a body. Regarding others as whole persons rather than as objects enables the basic energies of sexual attraction to remain free for genuine love: we can allow the sexual feelings to direct our selves toward a person whom we deeply respect. It is the perceived total worth of our spouse that calls us to intelligent abstinence. The conscious decision to abstain for good reason reminds us that our spouse has a mysterious total worth that calls for total regard.

> "We had to work through some things, like how we were using the method. And the idea of being 'available' during the infertile time was an issue. We had to get over the feeling we had to 'use' all the infertile days." Barbara Johnson

We would guess that boredom and the search for novel sexual thrills are rare among couples committed to practicing periodic abstinence because there is always a time to refrain from embracing, and to reflect. It requires discipline, communicating at many levels, and gradually leads to greater self- and mutual respect and joy.

Many couples liken periodic abstinence to the cultivation of courtship before a honeymoon each cycle. Others say that during pregnancy, when there is no family planning reason to abstain, the special benefits of periodic abstinence are "missed." And when some couples are faced with abstinence during pregnancy for the sake of their child, because of threatened miscarriage, their mutual continence is a great gift, disposing them as parents to receive with profoundest love each other and the child whom their selflessness will allow to see the light of day at birth.

It is true that abstinence dynamics sometimes illustrate the "forbidden" or "inaccessible fruit" syndrome: once denied, the attractiveness grows. Of course some couples complain about the abstinence time when they "can't have intercourse," but also don't seem to make use of the days when they "can." The situation calls for honest evaluation.

The time of abstinence is a time that couples can use to make a point to do things for each other, to expand the basis of their relationship instead of drawing apart, and to look ahead so a more relaxed atmosphere can be present when the infertile time comes. The couple may participate in a sports activity together or read a current book together and discuss it or either may enter the heart of the other by sharing a mutual interest, project, or hobby. It amounts to taking time to share life with each other. This is also a time to draw in a wider circle friends. The couple might make a special point to visit friends or to help others less fortunate in an effort to turn outward together beyond themselves. This need not happen only at the fertile time, but the time of abstinence does provide an occasion for growth not always tapped.

But Isn't This Just "Birth Control"?

First of all, NFP is family planning, in a positive sense. NFP educates a couple in human sexuality, including their fertility. Couples can use the NFP knowledge to achieve as well as avoid a pregnancy. Contraception, on the other hand, intervenes in bodily functions of the woman or in the act of intercourse, but only to avoid pregnancy. Using contraception gives the false impression that unintended pregnancy is really just the impersonal byproduct of contraceptive hardware malfunction, an infringement on one's life, rather than the natural outcome of freely chosen intercourse and a human person to be loved and nurtured.

"Openness to surprise is a deeply spiritual category intimately linked to acceptance of pain, yet without it life becomes stagnant and meaningless." Rhonda Chervin, philosophy professor Second, NFP is responsible child spacing. It does no harm to the husband's or wife's body, nor does it harm or destroy a developing child or endanger the life or development of a future child. Some methods of birth control result in complications which later make achieving a pregnancy difficult or even impossible. Some birth control measures can harm a newly conceived child if used while the woman is already pregnant. Others destroy life after conception — the IUD and virtually all hormonal contraceptives – at least possibly part of the time. They work by inducing a very early abortion. These cannot really be called "mere contraceptives."

In recent years some have started using the word "conception" to mean "implantation" (rather than "fertilization" — the union of sperm and egg). Why? So that the IUD and hormonal contraceptives can technically be called "contraceptives" rather than "abortifacients."[15,16] And so that people won't feel guilty about using them and causing early abortions.

As for sterilization, some say it simply does now what nature at menopause will surely do later. So why not get sterilized when your family size is reached? Well, there is a big difference between accepting the loss of fertility as opposed to mutilating a healthy organism. After all, suicide also does now what nature at death will surely do later! Suicide reflects hopelessness with life, as does sterilization with the power to give life.

NFP is an approach to family planning that proceeds from a hopeful attitude toward fertility: it is a human condition that can be understood and lived with in human fashion. And besides that, there are potential side-effects and irreversibility associated with surgical sterilization.

Once convinced about the value of NFP for health, interpersonal, and moral reasons, couples are interested in the scientific basis, effectiveness, and practical aspects of its use in their life.

> "Since using NFP, I have developed a persistent appreciation for sex. I've also observed that women who use NFP have better health than those who use the Pill and IUD." Jim Statt, M.D., OB/GYN

Challenges to NFP

Some find they have developed bad habits regarding sexual tension. They have learned to rely on sexual expression as a crutch to bolster their feeling of self-worth or as a way to control another person or to short circuit the relationship on a "physical level" to avoid sharing with another person on a deeper, intimate level. When sexual expression is seen as beyond one's control, help should be sought.

---

15. An article in *Contraception* (1994; 49:56-72) pointed to the abortifacient nature of the IUDs.
16. Larimore, W., Stanford, J., "Postfertilization Effects of Oral Contraceptives and Their Relationship to Informed Consent," *Archives of Family Medicine*, Feb. 2000 (http://archfami.ama-assn.org/cgi/content/full/9/2/126). Information regarding the Patch, NuvaRing, Seasonale, Lunelle, Depo-Provera, Norplant, and Jadelle indicates that these products affect the endometrium and possibly work as abortifacients.

Unresolved issues related to sex may surface, such as a past abortion or premarital sexual activity or a minor addiction to pornography or masturbation. Assistance and spiritual reconciliation need to be sought for one's personal peace of mind. There may have been a rape, or emotional or sexual abuse, and now there is difficulty trusting another sexually, even someone who is loved. Professional counseling is in order. Some people who have been sexually abused find that periodic abstinence as practiced in NFP provides a healing process. Periodic abstinence, freely chosen, out of love, enables them to develop trust and security with their spouse. There is a growing sense of specialness, acceptance, care, belonging, support, of feeling defended and safe — the very things one author says are needed to learn to love and to be loved.

How Shall We Speak of "Love"?

"Love" is overused and little understood. Some confuse feelings with love, believing that if they feel affectionate or sexually attracted or merely enjoy the presence of another, then the feelings are a measure of love for the other. Yet real love is a decision which may have little to do with one's emotions at any given moment. Eric Fromm speaks of love as knowledge, care, respect, and responsibility. St. Paul said it more robustly: "Love is always patient and kind; it is never jealous; love is never boastful or conceited; it is never rude or selfish; it does not take offense, and is not resentful. Love takes no pleasure in other people's sins but delights in the truth; it is always ready to excuse, to trust, to hope, and to endure whatever comes" (1Cor 13:4-7).

> "We need to understand the body language of sexuality. What do you want to say with a kiss? What does intercourse mean?"
> Rev. Marc Calegari, S.J.

In the end, love is a mystery — beyond complete human understanding. Real love is sacrificial love. Sacrificial love involves freely giving up something of oneself for the good of another. This is entirely distinct from what is called enabling the destructive behavior of another or maintaining a "victim" mentality. Perhaps time is given or self-centeredness mastered or one's initial dreams modified for the good of the family. Perhaps one stands by one's spouse in bad times, even when these times last for years. To be faithful, no matter what — here a hint is given of the Mystery which is God, the Mystery which is Love.

What Does the Catholic Church Teach about Marital Sexual Ethics?

Marriage and Family. The teachings are part of a larger vision of the nature and purpose of human life, which sees each person as made in the image and likeness of God. And thus, any way that God's unity, truth, goodness, and beauty manifest themselves in man or woman, there is a small but real reflection of the grandeur of God. When a couple desire to be one, pledge their fidelity, and anticipate marriage and family, a bit of the grandeur is made manifest again. From this union may come the procreation of a new human person, the transmission of the divine image, nurtured in time, destined for eternity—a matter involving God as well as the parents, and at the heart of human society. Given the dignity of the human person, each child conceived deserves a family and a societal environment supportive of the family.

> "We noticed positive changes in our relationship — better communication. Let's say contraception didn't impact on the intimacy sharing, but NFP did. As a husband, I had been through childbirth and I'd fought with the kids to use the bathroom. I couldn't imagine there was anything left sacred to talk about — but yes there was." Jeff Heinzen

Social by nature, the human person thrives only within a community setting. The family is the primary cell of society; the fate of the family and that of society are thereby closely intertwined. The family is also the primary cell of the Church and as such is a "mini-Church" (ecclesiola), called to be what the Church itself is as a whole: a sign and instrument of union with God and unity among humankind, giving hope and access to peace upon earth. The family is where people are loved not for what they have or can produce but simply because they are.

Family is the fruit of marriage, which is constituted by the marriage covenant. This covenant, if it be truly a marital covenant at all, requires a unitive disposition of lifelong fidelity and openness to parenthood. Sexual intercourse, properly called the marital act, belongs to marriage as a privileged expression of conjugal love and is honorable when it renews the marriage covenant as a chaste and intimate union respecting the inseparable connection between the unitive (love) and procreative (life) meanings of intercourse. This requires marital chastity.

Marital chastity means the proper integration of sexual inclination and activity within the whole picture of sacramental marriage "in the Lord." What makes Christian marriage "sacramental" is that it is consciously begun and lived as a sign and embodiment of the unshakable, fruitful union between God and his creation, and between Christ and the Church.

The Basic Principle. The superabundant generosity of God toward us (agape) is the foundation of the conjugal love in which marriage is to be lived and the criterion of its expression in genital sexuality. Thus, there is a "moral inseparability" of the unitive and the procreative meanings of the marital act by its very design and nature. This means that even though it is possible to separate the two meanings, it is wrong to do so. And engaging in genital activity while intentionally and actively intervening to separate the one or the other of these dimensions out is deemed immoral in relation to this principle. For instance, contraceptive measures are deemed morally defective in relation to this principle, but intercourse during a time thought to be infertile is morally acceptable, because there is respect for the natural disposition of the cycle of fertility.

> *Permitted:* Periodic abstinence for a good reason (e.g., illness, personal distress, need to avoid pregnancy) is of course permissible and proper, for no one is obligated always and everywhere to engage in intercourse, and no one may insist upon intercourse without due consideration for one's spouse and marital circumstance.
>
> *Not Permitted:* Objectively speaking, any chemical, mechanical, or surgical contraceptive sterilization, whether temporary or permanent, is wrong in relation to the principle of the moral inseparability of the unitive and procreative meanings of sexual activity, as is contraceptive intercourse itself. So, too, is any genital activity that is solitary (masturbation) or violent (rape) or extra-marital (fornication or adultery) or homosexual or anal or orgasmic oral-genital intercourse. Nocturnal emissions, being involuntary, involve no sin.

With regard to marital intimacies, the Church does not teach that the marital act is immoral if the spouses do not have simultaneous orgasm or if the wife fails to experience orgasm or if the husband fails to do so. Arousal and intimate caressing, including penetration, without orgasm, are permissible morally, though they may be frustrating psychologically. Likewise, during foreplay and afterplay, any kind of tender physical affection between spouses, mutually acceptable to them, is morally permissible, provided that any deliberate orgasm takes place in connection with the profound bodily union "in one flesh" of vaginal intercourse. Deliberate climaxing apart from undertaking to carry out such union, even by married couples, is wrong, a form of mutual masturbation, and to be avoided, because it, as well as the other types of unacceptable genital activity mentioned above, in the short or long run, ultimately undermines what the marital act is meant to be. The Church therefore emphasizes that the cultivation of chastity, having already begun in youth, is an indispensable aid to proper marital chastity.

> "I've had friends ask if I'm uncomfortable having intercourse with my wife without 'using' anything? I can't imagine anything else. NFP fulfills the goals we have in marriage: communication, faith, shared commitment, and family." Jerry Burchett

Theology of the Body.

Pope John Paul II revolutionized the Christian understanding of human sexuality with what has become popularly called "The Theology of the Body" and "The Theology of the Family." There are many excellent books, speakers, articles, and even online forums devoted to the topic. We urge you to explore the following websites to begin your journey:

http://www.theologyofthebody.net/index.htm,
http://www.nfpoutreach.org/Hogan_Theology_Body1.htm,
http://www.christopherwest.com/theologyofthebody.htm

Responsible Parenthood. Many assume that with the rejection of contraception no option is left to a couple but to have a baby every year. Those who have discovered NFP realize this is not true. On the other hand, some wonder whether there is a "formula" for the number of children a couple should have. There is not. But there are criteria for a discernment process that should be revisited from time to time: The couple is called to be generous and avoid a 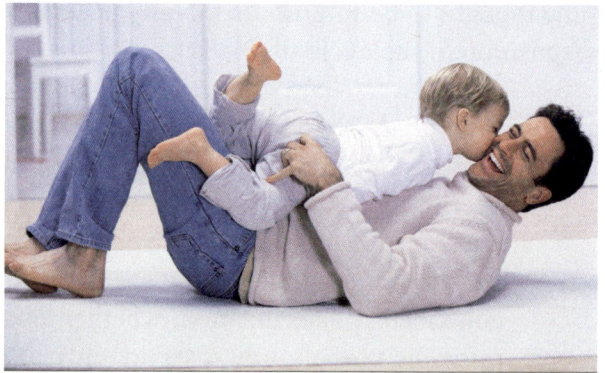 materialistic lifestyle, and to rear their children in a Christian lifestyle. They also need to take into account family and extended family obligations, social considerations, physical and psychological health, and financial matters. These factors need to be prayerfully considered, whether the couple is thinking of adding to their family or feeling inclined to forego temporarily or even permanently the joy of further children. The means of child spacing is to be moral (NFP), respecting the creative intention and role of God in each marital act.

Trouble Conceiving. Today couples are aware of methods for techniques which assist pregnancy, such as artificial insemination by husband or by a donor; surrogate motherhood by artificial insemination or by intercourse, or surrogate conception with embryo transplant; and in vitro fertilization.[17]

The first moral principle is that what is technically feasible is not by that fact morally or ethically permissible.

Second, the sole valid place for voluntary full genital activity is natural intercourse between husband and wife.

Third, though the desire for a child as an expression of a couple's love is natural, married couples do not have a "right" to a child, but only to the marital act — a child is a gift, to be received, as the fruit of love rightly expressed.

Bearing a child is a blessing, but not the sole or supreme one involved here. For marriage retains its value and indissolubility even when, despite the couple's intense desire for children, the couple is not blessed with any children. Is there perhaps another child somewhere, for whom their love, in God's providence, has been meant? Has adoption, foster parenting, or other ways to share your love been fully discussed and explored? Or another need, that only their love can address?

HIV/AIDS and Sexually Transmitted Diseases – A Concern. What about condoms for the marital act, should it be discovered that one spouse is HIV-positive? Can a marital act, rendered potentially life-threatening in such circumstances, really be an act of love? And even apart from the contraceptive matter of condom intercourse, can a couple endanger the life, safety, and security of any possible children, should pregnancy result from intercourse? Indeed, should not HIV/AIDS be considered a contraindication to any proposed marriage?

---

17. A 1987 Vatican document, *Donum Vitae* (Instruction on Respect for Human Life in its Origin and on the Dignity of Procreation) discusses these issues.

The matter of contraceptive intercourse has already been covered. With respect to the other issues, some physicians and ethicists, apart from Catholic sympathies, now find themselves, at least in the present state of knowledge regarding HIV/AIDS, maintaining that complete and continuous abstinence is the only responsible, ethical option open for a person who is HIV-positive.[18]

Science certainly supports prudence in the matter. For some of the most damaging sexually transmitted diseases (STDs) such as human papilloma virus, condoms have no preventive effect. The condom's efficacy over time with a variety of other STDs considering human behavior is suspect.[19] It is well known that the typical rate of pregnancy prevention for condoms for all U.S. women is 85 percent.[20] Concretely, that means that 15 out of 100 women will experience an unintended pregnancy when using a condom. Why would one expect greater success with respect to disease prevention when disease-carrying parasites, viruses, bacteria, and the like are considerably smaller than the sperm cell? For instance, the HIV virus is compared to a sperm in size what a football is to a football field!

But what about condoms and HIV/AIDS? There are conflicting reports, and the issues are complex to be sure. If condoms work, will people use them consistently and correctly every time? Even when the "partner" knows the other is HIV infected, apparently condoms are not used with the degree of frequency that is advocated. One study found 44 percent of the women "never used" or "not always" used the condom,[21] and another study found that 85 percent of the women "never," "rarely," or "sometimes" used a condom.[22] This data reflects usage by so-called "steady partners" or even married couples — adults with presumably strong emotional attachments to one another.

"Old fashioned morality," once ridiculed, is now being rediscovered as "common sense." Morality and the demands of public health coincide. A combination of virginity before marriage, monogamous fidelity within marriage, and NFP bring with them many benefits:
- Freedom from the negatives of out-of-wedlock pregnancy, for mother, for father, and for child.
- Freedom from physical damage from contraception or abortion.
- Freedom from HIV/AIDS or other sexually transmitted diseases.
- Freedom to develop fully your potential in human relationships.
- The best possible opportunity to achieve a pregnancy.

---

18. A concise and telling analysis of the conclusion that complete and continuous abstinence is the only responsible ethical option open to an HIV-positive person is provided by John Haas, PhD, STL in *Ethics and Medics* (March, 1991).
19. Fitch, J.T., "Are Condoms Effective in Reducing the Risk of Sexually Transmitted Disease?" *The Annals of Pharmacotherapy*, Sept. 2001.
20. Hatcher, R.A., et al, *Contraceptive Technology, Eighteenth Revised Edition*, Ardent Media, Inc., New York, 2004.
21. Saracco, A., et al, "Man-to-Woman Sexual Transmission of HIV: Longitudinal Study of 343 Steady Partners of Infected Men," *Journal of Acquired Immune Deficiency Syndromes*, vol. 6, no. 5, 1993.
22. Guimaraes, M., et al, "HIV Infection among Female Partners of Seropositive Men in Brazil," *American Journal of Epidemiology*, vol. 142, no. 5, 1995. Furthermore, this study found that of those who used a condom consistently 23% of the women converted to HIV positive within the year. Those who rarely/never used a condom and used oral contraceptives experienced a 55% seroconversion rate whereas those who never used a condom and did not use oral contraceptives experienced a 37% seroconversion rate. Data suggests that women using oral contraceptives have an increased risk factor for contracting HIV/AIDS (the actual reason is not fully understood because of the complexity of sexual behavior).

Isn't this kind of self-control only an ideal? It is indeed an ideal, and one possible and desirable of achievement by the grace of God. Actually, self-control or personal mastery is being seen anew, as a strength, not a stricture; as freeing, not constraining; as decisiveness, not negation. Far from being an unhealthy compulsivity to be in control, the mastery here at issue means personal vision, a focusing of one's energies, the cultivation of patience, an ability to see reality objectively, a gateway to positive development of one's potential. Translated into terms of NFP, these providential elements of the Church's moral vision are being seen as challenges worthy of our humanity.

Self-control may be experienced as difficult, but it is one of the fruits of the Spirit (Galatians 5:23). And the challenge of sexual self-mastery and marital chastity, far from destroying the spousal and parental dimensions of marriage, serves only to enhance and strengthen them. For conjugal love is a spiritual reality far more comprehensive than the marital acts in which it finds privileged expression. A pervading atmosphere of tenderness, respect, and consideration, together with marital chastity, allows the marital act to be truly honest and an occasion of spiritual joy.

> "When we were first married effectiveness was especially important to me. NFP works wonderfully for us. I taught for two years and then three months later became pregnant with our first child." Katie Jaeger

These seem like fine nuances. Is there really a difference between contraception and NFP? The difference between contraception and Natural Family Planning is much more than that of "different means" to the "same end":

> "It is a difference which is much wider and deeper than is usually thought, one which involves in the final analysis two irreconcilable concepts of the human person and of human sexuality. The choice of the natural rhythms involves accepting the cycle of the person, that is the woman, and thereby accepting dialogue, reciprocal respect, shared responsibility and self-control. To accept the cycle and to enter into dialogue means to recognize both the spiritual and corporal character of conjugal fidelity.

> "In this context the couple comes to experience how conjugal communion is enriched with those values of tenderness and affection which constitute the inner soul of human sexuality, in its physical dimension also. In this way sexuality is respected and promoted in its truly and fully human dimension, and is never 'used' as an 'object' that, by breaking the personal unity of soul and body, strikes at God's creation itself at the level of the deepest interaction of nature and person"— John Paul II, *Familiaris Consortio*, no. 32.

> "Spirituality is involved in NFP; you know that you're not abstaining alone. God is with you while you abstain, and you are abstaining for something good." Kent Purdy

Conscience. One could define conscience as the prospective practical judgment regarding a present course of action in relation to good and evil as understood by the person making the decision. In a broader sense it also includes retrospective evaluation of one's choices and reflection on the moral and ethical requirements of life worthy of the human subject and the human community. Ultimately, it includes as its most encompassing horizon, a religious perspective — for a Christian, one enlightened by revelation and faith. The Second Vatican Council spoke of conscience in *The Church in the Modern World*:

> "In the depths of his conscience, man detects a law which he does not impose upon himself but which holds him to obedience. Always summoning him to love good and avoid evil, the voice of conscience can when necessary speak to his heart more specifically: do this, shun that. For man has in his heart a law written by God. To obey it is the very dignity of man; according to it he will be judged.
>
> "Conscience is the most secret core and sanctuary of a man. There he is alone with God, whose voice echoes in his depths. In a wonderful manner conscience reveals that law which is fulfilled by love of God and neighbor. In fidelity to conscience, Christians are joined with the rest of men in the search for truth, and for the genuine solution to the numerous problems which arise in the life of individuals and from social relationships. Hence the more that a correct conscience holds sway, the more persons and groups turn aside from blind choice and strive to be guided by objective norms of morality.
>
> "Conscience frequently errs from invincible ignorance without losing its dignity. The same cannot be said of a man who cares but little for truth and goodness, or of a conscience which by degrees grows practically sightless as a result of habitual sin" — *Gaudium et Spes*, no. 16.

At the "core" of our being, an indestructible "spark" burns, where God "calls" us to an ever greater share in the unity, truth, and goodness of his own life. This "core" is "conscience" in its most basic manifestation of obligation: the "image" of God drawn to ever greater "likeness" to God, informed by a primordial intuition of a "communitarian sense of self" ordered towards the life of the Trinity as its final destiny. Conscience is thus "the Divine or Eternal Law" (God's own fulness of being as the norm of human existence) making itself felt within human experience as the "Natural Moral Law." Conscience does not legislate, but manifests this "law" as it "reveals" to us our true self, and the prior and objective inner requirements of human fulfillment. A maturing moral sense is thus said to discover (not invent) its imperatives, in conformity with which alone, happiness for the individual in community, and thus for each and for all, is to be found.

> **In practice, following one's conscience means a dynamic by which one will:**
> - Follow one's conscience (sincerity).
> - Continue to inform one's conscience (so it grows both true and certain).
> - Give the official teaching of the Church the benefit of the doubt, even when difficult.
> - If one finds oneself subjectively perplexed at the moment about assenting to the teaching, continue to pray and study to find a resolution in harmony with this teaching (otherwise one ceases to be in good faith).

Our choices in turn affect our moral perception. Attempting to "inform" our conscience can never be a matter of detached study while living the "low road": often it is a matter of saying, "I shall obey and thus come to understand." Luckily we find that doing what we please does not make us happy. It reminds us that

> "As I explored the deeper elements associated with family planning and sexuality, the rightness and beauty of the Church's teachings were very apparent." Beth Wells

moral truth in the end is something to be discovered (not something we invent). Christ tells us the very things we think will make us unhappy are those that lead us to true fulfillment (Mt 5:1-12, 10:38, 16:24 and parallels). We are prone to self deception, to our own destruction (cfr. Job 21:14, Is 5:20, Pr 17:15, Pr 12:15, 14:12 and 16:25, Jn 16:2, versus Ps 119:12,24 and Heb 10:22). Opinion polls don't count: "You shall not use the example of the many as an excuse for wrongdoing" (Ex 23:2).

How does this apply to non-Catholics? Some people humorously state that NFP does not mean "Not for Protestants." Many non-Catholics share this perspective, as they trace current social changes to their roots. Pro-life efforts have moved them to explore biblical and doctrinal issues related to sex, marriage, and family. They discover that "what God has joined together, let no man put asunder" applies to the marital act as well as to the marital covenant. Likewise they are becoming aware that the teaching of marital non-contraception was the common biblical Christian tradition until 1930, when the Anglican Lambeth became the first to allow the use of contraception in "hard cases." Christian lifestyle and contraception are ultimately seen as incompatible. Underlying all this is the belief that Christ gave Christians a new vision of what married life ought to be: a life of self-sacrificing love. Though such sacrifice may be difficult, love can make it easy, and perfect love can make it a joy. The traditional exhortation before marriage concludes with these words:

> "No greater blessing can come to your married life than pure conjugal love, loyal and true to the end. May, then, this love with which you join your hands and hearts today never fail, but grow deeper and stronger as the years go on. And if true love and the unselfish spirit of perfect sacrifice guide your every action, you can expect the greatest measure of earthly happiness that may be allotted to man in this vale of tears. The rest is in the hands of God. Nor will God be wanting to your needs; he will pledge you the life-long support of his graces in the holy sacrament which you are now going to receive."

> "Both the qualitative and quantitative data seem to indicate that the NFP couples have a stronger and more harmonious relationship with God than the contraceptive couples." Richard Fehring, DNSc

Passing It On

It is often said that the best gift parents can give their children is to love each other. In doing so, parents provide children with the environment they need to thrive. It is also known that what people do speaks louder than their words. In other words, in the area of sexuality the best advice a parent can give is his or her example. Children will form the basis of their sexuality during the first few years of life. The modeling parents provide is critical. Children who see parents that respect each other, treat each other with equality, and constructively work through their differences will learn a whole lot about sexuality that can never be read from a book.

> "My greatest reward as an NFP Provider is to see the way people react when they learn how the body works. They can see their fertility is positive." Janet McLaughlin

On a practical level, one good "side-effect" from practicing NFP is that it provides you with the ingredients for the "sexuality education" of your own children. When a couple understands their own reproductive anatomy and physiology and the generative process, and know and manage the expression of their own sexual feelings, they can communicate the multiple dimensions of married love to their children as needed. And there is a consistency between ideals held forth to the children and the way the parents live themselves.

There are attractive ways to inform young people or other adults about fertility, while forming a sense of self-worth, reverence, and responsibility. The example given earlier relating fertility to the seasons of the year is very useful and understandable.

If a seed is planted during the dry season, it will not germinate. But if planted during the wet season, there will be a harvest. And in between the dry and wet seasons, sometimes there's enough moisture for a seed to germinate.

The cervical mucus symptom, its relation to infertility and fertility during the cycle, and life and growth, are thus understandable as natural events. Young people can appreciate the story long before learning what the "seed" and "wet" and "dry" and so on mean in terms of NFP.

Accepting fertility is part of accepting oneself. As a young girl grows into a healthy woman, she needs to be able to understand her own development as something normal and good rather than as a disease to be treated. She needs the respect of the men in her life: her father, brothers, uncles, peer friends. According to Dr. Mary Ella Robertson, Professor of Social Policy at the Kent School of Social Work, Louisville, Kentucky, "The most important task that a girl faces is to learn to accept herself by accepting her own body. Knowledge of ovulation is indispensable if a girl is to succeed in self-acceptance. A girl must learn to live consciously with her cycle."

> In WINTER there is barren landscape (infertile dry days) and cool weather (low waking temperatures); the only growth occurring is silent, unseen, within the tree (initial growth of follicles and rebuilding of the uterine lining).
>
> Eventually SPRING (the fertile time) begins, with its rain (cervical mucus flow), the bursting of blossoms from their buds (ovulation of the egg from its follicle), and toward the end of spring, noticeably warming weather (temperature rise).
>
> The sun (the yellow body) makes SUMMER a season with warm, dry weather (high temperatures and dry days) and luxuriant foliage (enriched endometrium). There will be fruit (a baby) if the blossom (egg) was pollinated (fertilized).
>
> In AUTUMN the leaves fall (menstruation).

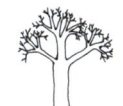 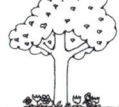 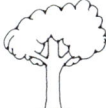 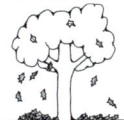

Resources

Abraham, G. E., has published extensively on PMS, see "Premenstrual Tension," *Current Problems in Obstetrics and Gynecology*, 3:1, 1980.

Ashley, B., and O'Rourke, K., *Health Care Ethics: A Theological Analysis*, 4th ed, St Louis, MO: Catholic Health Association, 1997.

Beck, A., *Love Is Never Enough*, New York: Harper Perennial, 1984.

Boys, G., "Natural Family Planning Client Survey," Portland, OR, 1985 (unpublished study of Western Oregon NFP clients 1982-1984, including Northwest Family Services clients).

Boys, G., *Natural Family Planning Nationwide Survey*, Final Report to the National Conference of Catholic Bishops, June 1989. A survey assessing NFP client satisfaction with the instruction and use of NFP and to determine the role of NFP in the couple relationship. This survey included 3,345 responses.

Elliott, P., *What God Has Joined...The Sacramentality of Marriage*, New York: Alba House, 1990.

Frank, P., and Raith, E., *Natürliche Familienplanung Physiologische Grundlagen, Methodenvergleich, Wirksamkeit—Eine Einführung für Ärzte und Berater* (Natural Family Planning: Physiological Foundations, Comparison of Methods, and Effectiveness—An Introduction for Physicians and Counselors), foreword by Gerd Döring, MD, Berlin: Springer-Verlag, 1985.

Fuller, R., Denman, H., and McLaughlin, J., *How to Teach the FACTS of Life*, Portland, OR: Northwest Family Services, 2000. A parent guide with practical tips on maturity, sexuality, communication, love, and relationships. The emphasis is the value of premarital abstinence.

Fuller, R. and McLaughlin, J., *Family Accountability Communicating Teen Sexuality*, Portland, OR: Northwest Family Services, 2002. Curricula for Middle School, Senior High and Parent Programs on sexuality, communication, love, relationships, and premarital abstinence, 1998. These are designed for public school settings.

Gallagher, A., Heinzen, A., Hogan, R., Taylor, R., *Teaching Catholic Family Values: A Parent Handbook*, Minnesota: Leaflet Missal Company, 1996.

Geerling, J.H., "Natural Family Planning," *American Family Physician*, vol. 52, no. 6, Nov. 1995.

Gottman, J., *Why Marriages Succeed or Fail*, New York: Simon & Schuster, 1994.

Grant, E., *Sexual Chemistry, Understanding Your Hormones, The Pill and HRT*, London: A Mandarin Paperback, 1995.

Gray, R. H., Kambic, R. T., "Epidemiological Studies of Natural Family Planning," *Human Reproduction*, February 1988.

Hartmann, C., *Science and the Safe Period*, 2nd ed, Baltimore: Williams and Wilkins, 1962.

Hatcher, Robert, et al, *Contraceptive Technology, 17th Edition*, New York: Irvington Publishers, Inc., 1998.

Herman, C., et al, *Periodic Abstinence in Developing Countries, Update and Policy Options*, United States Agency for International Development, Washington, DC, 1986.

Hilgers, T. W., *The Scientific Foundations of the Ovulation Method*, Pope Paul VI Institute Press, Omaha, NB, 1995.

Hilgers, T., et al, "Intermenstrual Symptoms and Ovulation," *Obstetrics and Gynecology*, August 1981.

Hogan, R., and LeVoir, J., *Covenant of Love: Pope John Paul II on Sexuality, Marriage, and Family in the Modern World*, Garden City, NY: Doubleday, 1985.

Huneger, R., and Fuller, R., *NFP Provider Education Guide*, 4th ed, Portland, OR, 1997 (privately printed).

Isaacs, D., *Character Building, A Guide for Parents and Teachers*, Ireland: Four Courts Press, 1984.

Jackson, R., "Ecological Breastfeeding and Child Spacing," *Clinical Pediatrics*, August 1988. *Breastfeeding and Natural Family Planning*, Selected Papers from the Fourth National and International Symposium on NFP, Chevy Chase, MD, November 1985.

John Paul II. A good starting point is *Familiaris Consortio*, 1981. "Theology of the Body" (1979-1981) talks are found in *Original Unity of Man and Woman* and *Blessed are the Poor of Heart*; see also *Reflections on Humanae Vitae* (July-November 1984). All four titles are published by Boston, MA: Daughters of St Paul. John Paul II's *Love and Responsibility*, San Francisco: Ignatius Press, 1981, is an updated English version of a work that appeared in 1960 in Polish.

Kambic, R. T., Martin, M. C., "Evaluating Client Autonomy in Natural Family Planning," *Advances in Contraceptives*, Sept. 1988.

Kass-Annese, B., Danzer, H., *The Complete Guide to the Treatment of Premenstrual Problems*, Los Angeles, CA: Patterns Publishing Co., 1984.

Kilpatrick, W., *Why Johnny Can't Tell Right from Wrong*, New York: Simon & Schuster, 1992.

Kippley, J., *Birth Control and the Marriage Covenant*, Cincinnati, OH: Couple to Couple League International, Inc., 1991 and *Birth Control and Christian Discipleship*, Cincinnati, OH: CCL International, 1985.

Kippley, J., and Kippley, S., *The Art of Natural Family Planning*, 4th edition, Cincinnati, OH: Couple to Couple League International, 1996.

Klaus, H., "Natural Family Planning: A Review," *Obstetrical and Gynecological Survey*, vol. 37, no. 2, 1982, 128-150. [Survey of biology, history, studies in NFP. Reply to Liskin report.]

Lanctot, C., et al, *Natural Family Planning Development of National Programs*, Washington, DC: International Federation for Family Life Promotion, 1984. [Summary of 1983 Hong Kong conference presentations.] *Abstracts of Papers Presented at the IVth Congress of the International Federation for Family Life Promotion*, Ottawa, Canada, 1986.

Lawler, R., Boyle, J., Jr, and May, W.E., *Catholic Sexual Ethics: A Summary Explanation and Defense*, Huntington, IN: Our Sunday Visitor, 1985.

Lee, J.R., et al, *What Your Doctor May Not Tell You About Menopause*, Warner Books, 1996.

Lee, J.R., et al, *What Your Doctor May Not Tell You About Premenopause*, Warner Books, 1999.

Lickona, T., *Character Matters*, New York: Touchstone Books, 2004

Lickona, T., *Educating for Character*, New York: Bantam Books, 1991.

Lickona, T., *Raising Good Children, From Birth Through the Teenage Years*, New York: Bantam Books, 1983.

Liskin, L.S., "Periodic Abstinence: How Well Do New Approaches Work?" *Population Reports*, Series I, Number 3, Baltimore: Population Information Program, September 1981.

McDowell, J., *Right from Wrong: What You Need to Know to Help Youth Make Right Choices*, Dallas, TX: Word Publishing, 1994.

Notarius, C., Markman, H., *We Can Work It Out*, New York: G.P. Putnam's Sons, 1993.

Paul VI, *Humanae Vitae*, 1968.

Pius XI, *Casti Connubii*, 1930.

Rodriguez-Garcia, R., et al, *Glossary of Natural Family Planning Terms*, Washington, DC: Institute for International Studies in Natural Family Planning, 1988.

Roetzer, J., *Family Size and Loving Marriage: A Guide to the Regulation of Conception* [Kinderzahl and Liebesehe. Ein Leitfaden zur Regelung der Empfängnis]. Herder: Vienna. 1965, 8 editions. *Natürliche Geburtenregelung: Der Partnerschaftliche Weg* (Natural Birth Regulation: Partnership in Family Planning). Herder: Vienna., First printing, 1979; 13th revised and expanded impression, 1985; new title since the 18th/19th printing in 1989 is *Natürliche Empfängnisregelung* (Natural Conception Regulation). Translated into numerous foreign languages. An expanded version, in English, from 1979 edition, appeared as *Family Planning the Natural Way*, Fleming H. Revell: NJ, 1981.

Roetzer, J., "Supplemented BBT and Regulation of Conception," *International Review of Natural Family Planning*, IV/1, Spring 1980, 1-18. [English version of Erweiterte Basaltemperaturmessung und Empfängnisregelung, Archiv für Gynäkologie, 206 (1968), 195-214, with author's 1979 updated notes on effectiveness.]

Roetzer, J., "The Sympto-Thermal Method: Ten Years of Change," *The Linacre Quarterly*, 45 (4), November 1978, 358-374.

Roetzer, J., Kaffanke, V., "Instruction Guide for the Taking of Magnesium," 1986. "The Therapeutic Effect of Magnesium in Dysmenorrhea," *Swiss Review of Medicine*, vol 79, no 16, 1990.

Shannon, M., *Fertility, Cycles, and Nutrition*, Cincinnati: Couple to Couple League International, Inc., 2001.

Sharma, R., Sevick, M.A., "Psychosocial Aspects of Natural Family Planning: A Review of Selected Literature," Washington, DC: Georgetown University, May 1990.

Shivanandan, M., *Challenge to Love*, Bethesda, MD: KM Associates, 1988. [Excerpt from Natural Sex, 1979.]

Smith, J.E., *Humanae Vitae, A Generation Later*, The Catholic University of America Press, 1991.

Taylor, R., Nerbun, A., *The Wonder of Me*, "Fertility Appreciation for Adolescents and Parents," Sumter, SC: DEPPA, 1999.

Taylor, R., Nerbun, A., Hogan, R., *Our Power to Love*, Sumter, SC: DEPPA, 2000.

Taylor, R., Theis, L., Easterday, M., *Awareness Wheel*, Wichita, KS: DEPPA of Kansas, 1996.

Truth and Meaning of Human Sexuality, Pontifical Council for the Family, 1995.

Vatican Congregation for the Doctrine of the Faith, *Donum Vitae*, 1987.

Vollman, R., *The Menstrual Cycle*, vol. 7, Philadelphia: W.B. Saunders Co., 1977. [A classic presentation of the menstrual cycle.]

Wilson, M., *Love and Fertility: the Ovulation Method, the Natural Method*, Family of the Americas Foundation, Inc., Mandeville, LA, 70470, 1986.

Glossary

Amenorrhea: Prolonged absence of menstrual periods.

Anovulatory: Without ovulation (a cycle without ovulation is anovulatory).

Basal Body Temperature (BBT): The temperature of the body at rest, unaffected by activity; taken upon waking (waking temperature).

Billings Method: See Ovulation Method.

Cervical Mucus: A mucous fluid secreted by crypts in the cervix.

Cervix: The lower, narrow part of the uterus — it opens at birth to provide a birth canal, and has mucus-producing "crypts."

Chastity: The virtue that allows us to do what is good and loving in the area of our sexuality. It includes refraining from sexual expression outside of marriage and remaining faithful to one's spouse in marriage, and respecting the unitive and procreative meanings in each and every act of sexual intercourse.

Conception: Initiation of a new human life and the process of pregnancy, beginning with fertilization of the woman's egg (ovum) by the man's seed (sperm).

Contraception: Interference with reproductive physiology or with the act of sexual intercourse in order to prevent conception. "Contraception" is to be distinguished from "Natural Family Planning" (which relies on natural fertility awareness and periodic abstinence when avoiding pregnancy) and from "Abortion" (destroying human life after conception to prevent birth).

Corpus Luteum: A gland which for 10-14 days after ovulation secretes the hormone progesterone. This gland is the remainder of the follicle (housing) from which the egg was released at ovulation, and it is yellow in color; hence, the name "corpus luteum" (Latin for "yellow body").

Endometrium: The inner lining of the uterus. It builds up each cycle to prepare for pregnancy and is discharged as menstruation if pregnancy does not occur.

Estrogen: A female hormone partly responsible for cyclic changes in the female reproductive system (unopposed estrogen causes the cervix to secrete mucus). It is also responsible for secondary sex characteristics in the woman.

Fallopian Tube: A tube, with a trumpet-like end, to receive and conduct the egg from either ovary to the uterus.

Fertile: Capable of conceiving a child.

Follicle: Any one of thousands of tiny containers each holding an ovum (egg). Upon releasing its ovum it becomes a gland called the "corpus luteum."

FSH: Abbreviation for "Follicle Stimulating Hormone," released by the pituitary gland in the brain to stimulate maturation of follicles in the ovary.

Full Thermal Shift Level: About 0.4° F above the pre-rise base (0.2° C or 0.36° F, to be exact).

Hormone: A glandular secretion influencing the action of cells in another part of the body.

Implantation: The process by which a newly conceived human being at the blastocyst stage imbeds itself in the lining of the uterus about 6-8 days after conception.

Infertility: The inability in a woman to conceive or in a man to fertilize an egg.

Lactation: Producing and yielding milk from the mammary glands (the breasts).

Lactational Amenorrhea Method (LAM): A method of family planning based on extensive evaluation of breastfeeding women around the world. When the following conditions are met, breastfeeding alone is 98 percent effective during the first six months after childbirth: no bleeding after 56 days postpartum and fully or near fully breastfeeding.

LH: Abbreviation for "Luteinizing Hormone," released by the pituitary gland in the brain to trigger ovulation.

Lochia: A blood and mucus discharge during the weeks after childbirth.

Luteal Phase: The time (normally 10-14 days) of significant progesterone secretion from the luteinized follicle or post-ovulatory corpus luteum before menses.

Menarche: The first menstruation (may occur before or after the first ovulation).

Menopause: The permanent cessation of menstruation and ovarian activity.

Menses (Menstruation): A blood and mucus discharge consisting of the sloughed-off outer layers of the uterus's inner lining (see True Menstruation).

Mittelschmerz: Intermenstrual pain; may be associated with ovulation.

Natural Family Planning (NFP): Knowledge about the fertility of the man and woman that enables the couple to achieve a pregnancy by uniting at the fertile time or avoid a pregnancy by refraining from intercourse and genital contact during the fertile time.

Os (os is Latin for "mouth"): The opening, or "mouth" of the cervix.

Ovary: The almond-shaped female reproductive organ containing the ova (eggs).

Ovulation: The process by which an ovum (egg) is released from its follicle (housing) through the wall of the ovary, making a woman temporarily fertile.

Ovulation Method (OM): The Ovulation Method of NFP developed by Drs. John and Lyn Billings of Australia to determine times of infertility and possible and probable fertility by exclusive reliance upon sensed and/or seen vulval manifestations of the absence, presence, traits, and changing or unchanging character of vaginal discharge, particularly of cervical mucus.

- -The World Organization of the Ovulation Method/Billings (WOOMB) was begun in 1977 to promote fertility awareness and family life through NFP according to the Billings Method.
- -Dr. Thomas W. Hilgers developed the Creighton Model of OM education based on the tissue-paper exam.

Ovum (plural "ova"): The woman's egg.

Peak Day: The final day of any sign of any trait of the "Most Fertile Sign" during a Possibly Fertile Time. During a typical mucus pattern the most fertile sign is EW-M; during a patch, M; during spotting, any bleeding; and during a prolonged discharge, any "difference" that may appear in the discharge. After each such "peak" a count of 1.2.3.4 days of fertility (until evening on the 4th) is assumed, in case ovulation was associated with it. If there is more than one peak in a cycle, the peak accompanied by a sustained temperature rise is considered the presumptively ovulatory peak of the cycle.

Post-ovulatory: The time of the cycle during which ovulation can no longer occur.

Postpartum: The time after childbirth.

Premature Ovarian Failure (POF): POF is a loss of ovarian function in women under 40. Periods stop, estrogen is low and the follicle stimulating hormone (FSH) level is elevated. Generally, it is said that the diagnosis requires at least 4 months without a period and two FSH tests, taken at least one month apart that are greater than 40 mIU/ML.

Premenopause: The time (usually the final 60 cycles or so) before menopause, during which the menstrual cycle pattern may change to reflect irregular, decreasing fertility by greater variation in cycle length, altered menstrual and cervical mucus patterns, fewer thermal shifts, and shorter luteal phases.

Pre-ovulatory: The time during the cycle prior to the occurrence of ovulation.

Pre-Rise Baseline: The highest undisturbed temperature of the final six "low" readings before the "thermal shift" (temperature rise). The amount of "rise" is measured from the Pre-Rise Baseline.

Progesterone: A female hormone secreted during the luteal phase to prevent further ovulation while enriching the uterine lining for possible implantation. It also causes the basal body temperature to rise and the cervical mucus to dry up.

Rhythm Method (Calendar Rhythm): A system of calculating the times of fertility and infertility in the present cycle on the basis of the length of previous cycles and certain assumptions about the time of ovulation and sperm survival. Rhythm was based on the independent but simultaneous discoveries of Ogino in Japan and Knaus in Austria in the late 1920's, that the post-ovulatory phase of the cycle is "constant" in length. It was gradually superseded by discoveries of specific hormonally-based signs of the possibly fertile time (the temperature, mucus, cervix, and secondary signs).

Sperm: Male sex cell that causes conception when it unites with a woman's egg.

Sympto-Thermal Method (STM): Any natural family planning system making use of all the signs of fertility: basal body temperature, cervical changes, cervical mucus, and various secondary signs. Some major NFP organizations providing Sympto-Thermal Method are: CLER (France), Dr. Roetzer (throughout German speaking world since 1951), SERENA (Canada since 1955), Couple to Couple League (1971), and Northwest Family Services (incorporated in 1983).

Thermal Shift: The change in basal body temperature level from early cycle lows to late cycle highs. The World Health Organization (W.H.O.) considers the shift to be "significant" for defining infertility after ovulation when the temperature rises within two days to "full thermal shift level" ($0.2°$ C/$.36°$ F or more above the highest of the final 6 lows) and stays there for three full days. The Sympto-Thermal Method requires crosschecking the temperature with cervix and/or mucus signs before assuming infertility, but because of the crosscheck, does not require such a pronounced temperature rise to evaluate the temperature pattern.

True Menstruation: Bleeding is only called "true" menstruation, for use with the 6-5 Day Rule, if the Basic Sympto-Thermal Rule was fulfilled prior to the onset of the bleeding.

Uterus: The womb, in which the baby grows during pregnancy.

Vagina: The soft muscular tract into which the man's penis fits during intercourse. The vagina connects the cervix with the vulva and is a birth canal.

Vulva: The outer parts of the female sex organs, including the vaginal lips (labia).

Index

6-5-0 Day Rule, 42
Abstinence, 1-2, 11, 34, 103-105, 109
Achieving (see assisted fertility; pregnancy)
Adolescence, 12
AIDS, 110-111
Anovulation (lack of ovulation)
    adolescence, 12
    premenopause, 12
    breastfeeding, 72
    stress, 40, 59, 64
    cycle pattern, 13
Arousal fluid, 47
Assisted fertility, 64-67
    medications, 61
    clomid, 65
    cycle pattern, 60-61
    morality, 63, 104
    progesterone, 61-63

Basal Body Thermometer, 16
Basal Body Temperature (see waking temperature) rule, 58

Basic Mucus Rule, 53-55
    after childbirth, 70-77
    continuous mucus, 55
    "Patch"Rule, 78
    post-hormone, 69-73
    premenopause, 82-84
Birth control pills, 69-71
Breast examination, 32, 95
Breast tenderness, 32
Breastfeeding, 74-79
    benefits, 74
    intensive, 76-77
    LAM, 78
    "Patch" Rule, 78

Catholic, 108-115
Cervical mucus
    arousal fluid, 47
    cervix, 28-31
    charting, 22-23
    continuous, 55, 70, 78
    Dry (Ø), 20

EW-M, 21
    factors which disturb, 18-19, 23, 56 88-90
    medications, 84-86
    pasty, 21
    "Patch" Rule, 78
    Peak Day, 25-26, 35-36, 53
    post-Peak stretch, 40-41
    premenopause, 82-84
    properties, 7-8, 20-22
    short mucus pattern, 48
    Sticky-M, 20-21
    tissue-paper examination, 19-23
    vaginal sensations, 24-26
Cervix, 7, 28-31, 34, 40, 45, 47
    charting, 30-31
    Peak Day, 30, 40
    post-intercourse discharge, 47
Chastity, 1, 3, 103-104
Christian, 108-113
Circadian body rhythms, 15, 18
Clomid, 65, 89
Clothing, 23
Completely Infertile Time, 9, 35-41, 55-58, 96
Conscience, 113
Contraception, 23, 58, 65-69, 86, 102-105
Digital thermometer, 16

"Ear" thermometer, 16
Earliest Sixth Last Low Rule, 49-52
Early Dry Days Rule, 45
Effectiveness, 96-97
    6-Day Rule, 96
    Completely Infertile Time, 96
    condoms, 11, 110
    Mucus-only, 96
    Relatively Infertile Time, 96
    Sympto-Thermal Rules, 35, 96
    Temperature Only Rules, 56
    use effectiveness, 92
Estrogen, 7, 24, 32, 93-94
    Hormone Replacement Therapy, 84, 86

Female anatomy and physiology, 6-8
Feminine hygiene, 23

Fertility appreciation, 103-106, 113
Five-Day Rule, 43-44

Genital herpes, 86
    cervix check, 86
Genital warts (see human papilloma virus)

History of NFP, 98-99
Hormones, 5-6, 34, 64, 90-91, 93-94
    estrogen, 7, 24, 32, 93-94
    progesterone, 7-8, 64, 71-72, 83, 93-94
    replacement therapy, 84, 86
Human papilloma virus (HPV), 29, 86
    cervical cancer, 86
    cervix check, 86

Intensive Breastfeeding, 76-77
Intercourse, 8, 34
Intermenstrual pain, 29-30, 32
Intermenstrual bleeding, 32, 34
    6-Day Rule, 42-44
    Basic Mucus Rule, 53
Intrauterine Device, 23, 69

Kegel exercises, 47
    arousal fluid, 47

Lactational Amenorrhea Method, 78
Love, 1, 103, 105
Luteal phase, 13, 50, 59, 63, 95

Male anatomy and physiology, 5-6
Mean Temperature Rule, 56-58
Menopause, 12, 13, 82
Menstruation, 9-10, 12, 34, 94-95
    length, 10
    missing period, 55
    myths, 94-95
    non-menstrual bleeding, 32, 43, 81
    phases, 9-10, 12
    reproductive categories, 13
    stress, 59
    true menstruation, 41, 42, 74
Minerals, 87
    premenopause, 82

    premenstrual syndrome, 85
Miscarriage, 75
"Missed" period, 55
Mucus (see Cervical Mucus)

Natural Family Planning
    after childbirth, 74-81
    breastfeeding, 74-79
    charting, 15-34
    effectiveness, 96-97
    marriage enrichment, 1-3, 103-115
    post-hormone, 69-73
    premenopause, 82-84
Natural progesterone, 64, 66

Osteoporosis, 84
    alternatives to HRT, 84
    premenopause, 84
Ovulation, 6-9, 93-95

Peak Day, 25-26, 35-36, 53
    cervix, 30, 40
    post-Peak stretch, 40-41
    Sympto-Thermal Rule, 35-41
Penis, 5
Possibly Fertile Time, 10
Post Depo-Provera, 71-72
Post-IUD, 73
Post-Pill/Patch, 70-71
Post-implant, 73
Post-intercourse discharge, 47
    arousal fluid, 47
    Kegel exercises, 47
Pregnancy, 61-67
    aids, 65
    clomid, 65
    due date, 61
    post-pill, 70-71
    scant mucus, 64
    sex selection, 61
    short luteal phase, 64
Premenopause, 12, 13, 82-84, 86
    osteoporosis, 84
    remedies, 84
Premenstrual Syndrome (PMS), 85

remedies, 85
    symptoms, 85
Progesterone, 7-8, 64, 66, 71-72, 83, 93-94
Relatively Infertile Time, 10, 41-55
Reproductive categories, 12
Responsible parenthood, 110
Scrotum, 5
Secondary signs, 31-32
Seminal fluid, 5, 46-47
Sensations (see vaginal sensations)
Short cycles, 42-44, 48
Shortcut approach, 52
Six-Day Rule, 42-44, 56
Sperm, 5-6
Sterilization, 106
Stress, 40, 55-57, 64, 85
Sympto-Thermal Rule, 35-41

Talcum powder warning, 23
Temperature, 15-19, 35-41, 54-57
The "Shot," 71-72
Thermometers, 16
Thyroid, 64, 87
Tissue-paper exam, 19-23
    EW-Mucus, 21
    Sticky M, 20-21
    Tissue dry (Ø), 20
    traits, 22
    wipe-look-test, 19-20
Toxic shock syndrome (TSS), 86

Uterus, 6

Vagina, 6-7
Vaginal sensations, 24-26
    dry (d), 24
    moistness ( ), 24
    lubrication (L), 24
Vitamins, 59, 61, 64, 81, 84-85, 87-88, 90
    m
    M
Waking temperature, 15-19
    basal body thermometer, 16
    biphasic pattern, 13
    "ear" thermometer, 16
    consistency, 18
    digital thermometer, 16
    disturbances, 18-19, 56
    encircled temperatures, 37-38
    evenings or rotating shift, 18
    Full thermal shift level, 37
    Pre-Rise Baseline, 36-38, 56
    rapid rise, 35
    shallow rise, 35
    six low temperatures, 36-39, 46, 49-51
    short cut approach, 52
    spare thermometer, 17
    techniques, 16-17

Yeast infection, 55, 58